"John Geyman, in his book, *How Obamacare Is Unsustainable: Why We Need a Single-Payer Solution for All Americans*, really gets it. He artfully describes how we have arrived in the mess we find ourselves, explains the underlying pathologies in our health care system and politics that have led us here, and clearly describes the only rational, evidence-based way out. A must read for anybody interested in understanding our current health care dilemma and the best way to fix it."

—Phillip Caper, M.D., internist with long experience in national health policy work dating back to the early 1970s, past chairman of the National Council on Health Planning and Development, and founding member of the National Academy of Social Insurance

"A brilliantly clear account of how the Affordable Care Act—or Obamacare—emerged in 2010 legislatively and has since then confronted, with great difficulty, the problems of insuring those without health coverage. I can think of no book that competes with Geyman's in explaining this complicated subject."

—Ted Marmor, Ph.D. professor emeritus of public policy and management at Yale University, author of *The Politics of Medicare*, co-author of *Social Insurance: America's Neglected Heritage and Contested Future*, and member of the Institute of Medicine.

"This important book provides a vivid, data-driven critique of the Affordable Care Act, describing how the new law accentuates many of the ills it was designed to correct. Thus, despite the ACA's good intent, we still have soaring costs, unequal access to care, and a health care system where materialism dominates moral commitment and the drive for profits trumps the needs of patients at every turn. The book also provides a passionate argument for a single-payer system. A major contribution to the debate about the future of health care in America."

—Kenneth Ludmerer, M.D., professor of medicine and history at Washington University in St. Louis, author of *Time to Heal*, and past president of the American Association for the History of Medicine

Also By John Geyman, M.D.

The Modern Family Doctor and Changing Medical Practice

Family Practice: Foundation of Changing Health Care

*Family Practice: An International Perspective in Developed Countries
(Co-Editor)*

Evidence-Based Clinical Practice: Concepts and Approaches (Co-Editor)

Textbook of Rural Medicine (Co-Editor)

Health Care in America: Can Our Ailing System Be Healed?

*The Corporate Transformation of Health Care:
Can the Public Interest Still Be Served?*

Falling Through the Safety Net: Americans Without Health Insurance

Shredding the Social Contract: The Privatization of Medicare

The Corrosion of Medicine: Can the Profession Reclaim its Moral Legacy?

*Do Not Resuscitate: Why the Health Insurance Industry is Dying,
and How We Must Replace It*

*Hijacked: The Road to Single Payer in the Aftermath of
Stolen Health Care Reform*

*Breaking Point: How the Primary Care Crisis
Endangers the Lives of Americans*

The Cancer Generation: Baby Boomers Facing a Perfect Storm
Second Edition

*Health Care Wars
How Market Ideology and Corporate Power Are Killing Americans*

*Souls on a Walk:
An Enduring Love Story Unbroken by Alzheimer's*

HOW OBAMACARE IS UNSUSTAINABLE

Why We Need a Single-Payer Solution For All Americans

John Geyman, M.D.

Copernicus Healthcare
Friday Harbor, Washington

How Obamacare Is Unsustainable:
Why We Need a Single-Payer Solution For All Americans

John Geyman, M.D.

Copernicus Healthcare
Friday Harbor, WA

First Edition

Book design, cover and illustrations by W. Bruce Conway
Author photo by Anne Sheridan

softcover: ISBN 978-0-9887996-9-1

Library of Congress Control Number: 2014957666

Copernicus Healthcare
34 Oak Hill Drive
Friday Harbor, WA 98250

www.copernicus-healthcare.org

Dedication

To the many millions of Americans who suffer under the burdens of our failing profit-driven health care system—may your voices be heard and your needs for care be met.

Contents

Part Three:
The Single-Payer Alternative: National Health Insurance

TABLES AND FIGURES

Acknowledgments

The support and encouragement of many colleagues have made this book possible. I am indebted to many others, as cited in references throughout the book, for their work advancing our better understanding of the Affordable Care Act over its five-year experience amidst our changing health care system. I especially appreciate the constructive comments of these colleagues for their reviews of selected chapters:

- Dr. Don McCanne, family physician and Senior Health Policy Fellow for Physicians for a National Health Program
- Dr. David Gimlett, family physician and former Medical Director of Inter Island Medical Center in Friday Harbor, Washington
- Mark Almberg, director of communications for Physicians for a National Health Program

Many sources of reference materials were helpful as this book came together, including reports from the Centers for Medicare-Medicaid Services, the Center for Studying Health System Change, the Commonwealth Fund, the Congressional Budget Office, the Economic Policy Institute, the General Accounting Office, Healthcare-NOW!, the Kaiser Family Foundation, the Medicare Rights Center, the National Bureau of Economic Research, the Office of Inspector General, the Organization for Economic Cooperation and Development, Physicians for a National Health Program, and Public Citizen. Thanks also to the publishers, journals, and cartoonists who granted permission to reprint or adapt materials as cited in the book.

As with all previous books with Copernicus Healthcare, W. Bruce Conway has again done a stellar job of book design, cover and interior layout, preparation of graphics, and typesetting. Thanks to Carolyn Acheson of Edmonds, Washington, for her professional reader-helpful indexing of the book. And most of all, I am grateful to Emily Geyman, my new bride, for her encouragement, suggestions, eagle eye in editing/proofing, and promotion of the book.

PREFACE

The Inconvenient Truth about Obamacare

As we all know, the intense debate over Obamacare, or the Affordable Care Act (ACA), is a polarizing issue that sharply divides political parties and the public. Confusion reigns over its benefits, problems and prospects as claims and counterclaims fill press and media coverage. As both political parties attempt to gain advantage over the issue, hard, unbiased information is hard to come by. Instead we see smoke and mirrors as warring interests attempt to move the debate to their side of the argument.

And as we also know too well, health care in this country has become unaffordable and inaccessible to many tens of millions of Americans who too often are bankrupted by any major illness or accident. Our supposed "safety net" of public programs are underfunded and falling apart, with many politicians on the right cutting them further in the name of austerity. Conservatives tell us to take more personal responsibility for our own health care—tough luck if we can't afford it. Most Democrats find themselves loyally trying to defend the ACA as President Obama's signature legislative success, arguing that the initial website's glitches were just bumps on the road to a successful outcome and that we should stay the course. Across the political chasm, Republicans are finally giving up on repealing the law, but seek to kill it with a thousand cuts while offering no new ideas of their own.[1] Meanwhile, corporate stakeholders in our medical-industrial complex are thriving, Wall Street is happy, and health care stocks are soaring.

This book is an attempt to make sense out of all this—to cut through the rhetoric, disinformation and myths to assess what is good and bad about the ACA, and to ask whether or not it can remedy our system's four main problems—uncontrolled costs, unaffordability, barriers to access, and mediocre, often poor quality of care. We are now roughly at the halfway point in the legislative life of the ACA, so we have a full five years' experience to assess. Many supporters of the bill will say that it is too early to declare the ACA dead, and that we should let it run its full course. My point is that we already know how it will end—inconvenient truth as that may be for its architects and supporters—and what comes next is the real question.

As you will see, the ACA does not survive an objective look at its prospects. I will make the case that it is fatally flawed by political compromises along the way, as described in an earlier book, *Hijacked: The Road to Single-payer in the Aftermath of Stolen Health Care Reform.*[2] So where do we go now as the middle-class withers away, inequality increases, public confidence in politicians and government is at an historic low, and as the future of the American dream is called into question for much of the population?

Health care reform has a long and turbulent history in this country. In Part One, we will briefly trace historical roots of various reform attempts over the years, and summarize some of the major trends that have changed the delivery system, professional roles and values, the ethics of health care, and the role of government vs. the private sector. In Part Two, we will compare the ACA's promises with realities of what it has accomplished, examine its initial outcomes on access, cost containment, affordability and quality of care, ask whether its flaws can be fixed with a private insurance industry, and point out the lessons that we can already take away from the first five years of the law. In Part Three, we will discuss the many myths that are perpetuated by opponents of single-payer national health insurance (NHI) and show how that approach stands ready to deal directly with what has become a national disgrace—our increasingly fragmented and cruel health care system that serves corporate interests at the expense of ordinary Americans. We will make the case for NHI in three ways—economic, social/political, and moral. Most other advanced countries around the world came to this conclusion many years ago.

Why this book now? With the 2014 midterm elections behind us, divisions between the parties are even more polarized. The future of health care is even more uncertain. The 2016 election cycle is already underway, and both parties have to confront the failures of yet another incremental attempt to reform our so-called health care system. We have a short year and a half to re-assess where we are and try once again to get health care reform right. As much of the public knows all too well, the stakes get higher every day.

This book will necessarily deal with two closely intertwined subjects—the financing and delivery systems of U.S. health care. Since the financing and the flow of money determines most of what happens on the delivery side, we will focus our attention in the opening chapter to previous efforts to enact national health insurance. As you will soon see, this goes back 100 years.

John Geyman, M.D.
Friday Harbor, WA
January, 2015

References

1. Weisman, J. With health law cemented, GOP debates next move. *New York Times*, December 26, 2013.
2. Geyman, JP. *Hijacked: The Road to Single-payer in the Aftermath of Stolen Health Care Reform*. Monroe, ME. Common Courage Press, 2010.

Part One

HISTORICAL BACKGROUND

"The only thing new in the world is the history you don't know."[1]

—President Harry Truman

1. As quoted by Stevens, RA. *History and Health Policy in the United States*. New Brunswick, NJ. Rutgers University Press, 2006, p. 5.

CHAPTER 1

A CENTURY-LONG STRUGGLE
OVER HEALTH INSURANCE

The time is present when the profession should study earnestly to solve the questions of medical care that will arise under various forms of social insurance. Blind opposition, indignant repudiation, bitter denunciation of these laws is worse than useless; it leads nowhere and it leaves the profession in a position of helplessness as the rising tide of social development sweeps over it.[1]

The battle over health insurance in the U.S. is a long story going back more than 100 years. The above statement was made by the social insurance committee of the American Medical Association in 1917, and its final report favoring health insurance was actually approved by the AMA House of Delegates that year.[2] Theodore Roosevelt had campaigned for national health insurance as a presidential candidate with the Progressive Party in 1912, and there appeared to be a movement toward a national plan. Congress held hearings on the matter in 1916, and fifteen states, including New York, Massachusetts and California, introduced compulsory health insurance bills between 1916 and 1920.[3]

Despite the AMA committee's call to take leadership on the issue, its own state chapters soon weighed in with strong opposition to any system of national health insurance. The AMA reversed its policy, even closing down its own committee on social insurance. Ever since, the AMA has been a constant reactionary opponent of any such plan. Although only about one in five U.S. physicians are members of the AMA today, it is still a powerful lobby for the status quo and its own independent prerogatives.

In 1917, the U. S. was already lagging behind nations in Europe in developing one or another form of national health insurance. Ten European countries had done so between 1883-1913. Germany had led the way with compulsory sickness insurance for workers, covering medical care as well as benefits for lost wages during periods of illness. Other countries later followed with similar national plans, including Austria in 1888, Hungary in 1889, Norway in 1909, Britain in 1911, Russia in 1912, and the Netherlands in 1913. Other variations of sickness insurance were being developed during those years in France, Denmark, Sweden, Switzerland, and Italy.[4]

Despite early momentum toward health insurance in some states and in Congress, the issue was soon eclipsed by other events as the country entered World War I in 1917. National priorities changed abruptly, and the idea of compulsory health insurance became viewed as a foreign idea, tarnished as un-American by its early connections with Germany. Four more major attempts to establish national health insurance would follow over the next 100 years, the next to reappear during the Depression years.[5]

Historians have drawn some interesting conclusions about why health insurance had so much difficulty gaining traction during that Progressive era. Together with Lloyd George and Winston Churchill in England, Theodore Roosevelt had been a strong supporter of social health insurance, but he was defeated by Woodrow Wilson in 1912. The three strongest opponents of social health insurance in this country—organized medicine, labor and business—each fought it for different reasons. In his landmark book, *The Social Transformation of American Medicine*, Paul Starr concluded that ideology, historical experience and the overall political context played the largest role in shaping how groups identified and expressed their interests. Many opponents worried that compulsory insurance would undermine individual initiative and self-reliance. Medical societies worried about threats to their incomes, autonomy, and dealing with an enlarging bureaucracy. Remarkably, the AFL opposed compulsory health insurance, with its president, Samuel Gompers, denouncing it as an unnecessary, paternalistic reform that would create a system of state supervision of peoples' health. Business leaders generally rejected the argument that health insurance would add to productive efficiency.[6]

The first defeat of compulsory health insurance in America carried with it some surprising ironies as compared to England and Germany. While compulsory health insurance in this country was viewed as antithetical to the American spirit of independence and individualism, it was brought forward in England and Germany by already powerful central governments, both for defensive reasons that were somewhat different for each. In Germany, Bismarck faced a growing challenge from the Social Democratic Party. After outlawing the Party, he went further in seeking a "welfare monarchy" to assure workers' loyalty.[7]

In England, Lloyd George wanted to increase industrial productivity, create a healthier workforce and military, and decrease class unrest by bringing workers into an expanded welfare system; as he said at the time, "You cannot maintain an A-1 empire with a C-3 population."[8]

Both Germany and England were using social insurance against the cost of illness as a way of "turning benevolence to power."[9] These examples are in sharp contrast with the defeat of compulsory health insurance in the U.S. during the Progressive era, when our country had a comparatively weak and divided government.

Second Attempt to Enact National Health Insurance (NHI): 1932-1938

Concern was growing during the 1920s over the increasing costs of medical care, especially of hospitalization. Various experiments were taking place around the country to develop prepaid insurance. Local physician groups in some areas took the lead in setting up various kinds of insurance plans. Workmen compensation programs had been established in 37 states by 1919.[10] As the country entered the Great Depression in 1929, hospitals were in dire straits, with more than one-third of general hospital beds unfilled. One such hospital, Baylor's University Hospital in Dallas, Texas, designed and implemented a prepaid group hospital plan for more than 1,300 Dallas teachers. That became the prototype for later Blue Cross plans.

As the Depression deepened in the 1930s, many other prepaid group insurance plans were developed across the country for both hospital and medical care. A landmark report by the Committee on the Costs of Medical Care (CCMC), a group of 50 economists, physicians, public health professionals, administrators and scholars, was released in 1932 calling for promotion of group practice and *voluntary* prepayment plans.[11] The report was immediately attacked by Dr. Morris Fishbein, then editor of *The Journal of the American Medical Association,* as "socialism and communism, inciting to revolution."[12]

Another important report at the time was that of the Committee on Economic Security, which led to the Social Security Act of 1935. It endorsed the principle of national health insurance. Meanwhile, Blue Cross was promoting itself as an alternative to compulsory health insurance, arguing that it would:

> *Eliminate the demand for compulsory health insurance and stop the reintroduction of vicious sociological bills into the state legislature year after year—Blue Cross Plans are a distinctly American institution, a unique combination of individual initiative and social responsibility. They perform a public service without public compulsion.*[13]

Although President Franklin D. Roosevelt supported the concept of national health insurance, he decided not to take on the strong opposition of organized medicine. The Social Security Act became law in 1935 without any provision for NHI. While the federal government did further consider "a general medical care program supported by taxes, insurance, or both," over the next three years,[14] FDR decided in 1938 to leave the issue until a future campaign.

Third Attempt to Enact NHI: 1945-1950

The failure to enact national health insurance during the New Deal years left a policy vacuum that was soon filled with joint efforts by the American Hospital Association and Blue Cross plans to support not-for-profit insurance plans. FDR, however, returned the issue of NHI to his legislative agenda in his 1944 State of the Union message, asking Congress for an "economic bill of rights", including a plan for adequate medical care.[15]

FDR did not live to follow up on this agenda. After his death in 1945, President Harry Truman proposed a comprehensive NHI program the next year, to be administered through the Social Security system, with its basic provisions incorporated into the Wagner-Murray-Dingell bill in Congress. Truman assured critics that "people will get hospital and medical services just as they do now and that the program would not be socialized medicine." However, opponents quickly responded with a strong and successful lobbying effort, led by the American Medical Association (AMA) and the American Hospital Association. In a political climate marked by the public's neo-Cold War fears of "socialism", the bill soon died in a congressional committee of a Republican-controlled Congress.[16] The only success from this defeat was an amendment to the Social Security Act passed in 1950 whereby federal "vendor payments" could be made to states as matching funds for medical care of welfare recipients. That would reappear 15 years later with the enactment of Medicaid.[17]

True to form once again, the AMA battled against NHI, arguing for voluntary insurance with a vehement campaign of distortion, arguing that a compulsory national plan "would bring socialism and turn physicians into slaves."[18] This time the opposition was joined by other interests, including the American Bar Association, the Chamber of Commerce, large corporations, and most of the country's press.

An interesting and little-known sidelight to the history of attempts to enact universal health insurance took place in California during the World War II years. Governor Earl Warren, elected to three terms in 1942, 1946 and 1950, called for a compulsory statewide system of health care. In his January 1945 inaugural address, he said:

> *[that he was] sure that the cost of medical care could be reduced 'without injuring anyone' and that it would 'relieve millions of our people from the spectre of bankruptcy and*

*indigency which are the present-day results of the cost of
illness.'[19]*

Republicans across the state soon attacked the proposal and
stated their unalterable opposition to the "socialization or regi-
mentation of labor, industry, business or the professions under
any guise or subterfuge whatsoever."[20] The proposal never saw
the light of day as Governor Warren was appointed by President
Dwight Eisenhower to become the 14th Chief Justice of the United
States.

Fourth Attempt to Enact NHI: 1973-1974

Politics over the simmering issue of health insurance became
more complicated after 1950. Mark Peterson, a leading policy analyst and scholar in government affairs, has described the increasing polarity between competing interests in terms of *stakeholders*
(interests that benefit from the status quo) and *stake challengers*
(interests that challenge the status quo because they either do not
benefit or are harmed by it). As applied to U.S. health care, Peterson notes that a homogeneous group of major stakeholders, especially the AMA, American Hospital Association, and the health
insurance industry, were not confronted by serious stake challengers from 1890 to the 1950s.[21]

The political dynamic was soon to change. Health insurance
for the elderly was a big issue during the presidential elections of
1960 and 1964, culminating in the passage of Medicare in 1965 as
the nation's first compulsory health insurance program covering
ten percent of the population. Medicaid was enacted at the same
time as a joint effort with the states, with eligibility varying widely from state to state. A growing coalition of stake challengers was
gaining momentum, and debate was growing over whether health
care should be a right. The U.S. Supreme Court even recognized
"an acknowledged right to health derived from a constitutionally
guaranteed right to life and happiness."[22]

Democrats controlled Congress in 1970 as the Nixon administration found itself facing various liberal initiatives, including a

single-payer proposal by Senator Ted Kennedy. President Nixon countered with his own "Play or Pay" health care proposal whereby employers would either offer acceptable health insurance coverage to their employees or pay a tax that would finance coverage from an insurance pool that would also cover the unemployed.[23]

A National Health Insurance Standards Act would be established, together with a federally administered Family Health Insurance Program to provide a basic benefit package for low-income families. The Nixon plan also called for widespread adoption of health maintenance organizations (HMOs) with the hope to cover 90 percent of the population by 1980.[24] Nixon had moved beyond a traditional conservative agenda by recasting some liberal ideas.

A polarized debate in Congress led to a compromise proposal, the Kennedy-Mills bill, which would have required co-payments of 25 percent and assured that no individual or family would have paid more than $1,000 for health care in any one year. As the political process became diverted by Vietnam and the Watergate scandal, however, bipartisan support of Kerr-Mills could not be gained, and that effort toward national health insurance went the way of its predecessors. Reflecting on this defeat in his 1982 book, Paul Starr had this to say:

If the name on the administration's plan had not been Nixon and had the time not been the year of Watergate, the United States might have had national health insurance in 1974.[25]

Fifth Attempt to Enact NHI: 1993-1994

U.S. health care became rapidly corporatized during the 1980s and 1990s in a growing market filled by for-profit health plans, hospital chains and other organizations. Managed care was taking hold in a new world of HMOs, physician-hospital associations, and independent practice associations. Many Blue Cross plans converted to for-profit status, announcing a goal to provide 90 percent of their benefits through managed care contracts by the year 2000. Competition was intense as costs increased, access decreased, and unpredictable quality became common within the fast-changing health care landscape.[26]

Health care reform was again a hot issue during the 1992 presidential election cycle. Although most of us will not recall, five different NHI proposals were brought forward in Congress.

The American Health Security Act (Clinton Health Plan) attracted the most attention. From the beginning, Hillary Rodham Clinton's Health Care Task Force was carefully selected to represent the major stakeholders in the medical-industrial complex. They were deeply divided among themselves, each pursuing their own self-interest. Big business, for example, supported employer mandates, while small business rebelled against that requirement. The goals of large insurers had little in common with small insurers. The fight over the Clinton Health Plan (CHP) was so intense that it never got out of committee to a vote on the House floor. These two post-mortem assessments tell the story:

> *The CHP's fatal flaw, at least in these terms, lay in its attempt to combine employer mandates (which attracted health interests and repelled many employers) and cost control (which attracted employers and repelled health interests). This pairing made for a slow dance to the right, as reaction set in from all quarters against employer mandates, against spending controls, against any increased federal presence in health care.* "[28]
>
> —Professor Colin Gordon, professor of history at the University of Iowa

> *Every special interest in the health industry—big insurance companies and middle-sized ones, the managed care industry, employers who provide health benefits and those who do not, big corporations and small business, hospitals, and physicians—rolled into Washington, D.C., with fat bankrolls and slick lobbyists.*[29]
>
> —Charles Andrews, author of *Profit Fever: The Drive to Corporatize Health Care and How to Stop It*

Lost in the shuffle and virtually uncovered by the media, the bill sponsored by liberal Democrats—Rep. Jim McDermott's (D-WA) Single-payer bill (H.R. 1200)—was the only proposal of the five alternatives to have grassroots support and attract the largest number of supporters in Congress. Modeled after the Canadian system with public financing and a private delivery system, it was the only one of the five to pass out of committee. It was marginalized by the major media and even ridiculed as "extreme" or "utopian."[30] ABC's *World News Tonight* mentioned it only once in all of 1993.[31]

It is also interesting to compare the two bills offered by the GOP leadership in the House and Senate—some provisions are part of Republican ideas today while others, accepted then, are rejected and hard-fought as more liberal ideas.

The demise of the highly publicized CHP was a political disaster for the Clinton administration, at least partly responsible for heavy losses by the Democrats to the Republicans in the 1994 midterm elections. Blame was widely circulated. After all the political compromises along the way, it was widely seen as far too complex, too expensive and poorly conceived. These perceptions illustrate why it never got off the ground:

Clinton's plan rests on the belief that an army of policy wonks can predict what would happen under a program that would change one-seventh of the economy, which 30 years of experience tells us we can't do.[32]

—Joseph Califano, secretary of health, education and labor in the Carter administration

The might of the anti-reform power brokers literally blocked definitive consideration of the single-payer proposal. This was possible only because President Clinton, from the outset, acknowledged the superiority of this alternative while signaling his conviction that it was infeasible. That is, he lacked the political will to confront the powerful opponents and the political honesty to admit that his "mandated premiums" were as much of a tax as the progressive tax base of single-payer. In the end, it was the fatally flawed CHP that was so infeasible it could not even get out of Committee![33]

—Quentin Young, M.D., national coordinator
for Physicians for a National Health Program

The United States is the only country where the welfare state is, for the most part, privatized. Consequently, when workers lose their jobs, health care benefits for themselves and their families are also lost. In no other country does this occur. This is why the corporate class and its instruments in the United States oppose establishing government-guaranteed universal entitlements. They strengthen the working class and weaken the capitalist class. The staggering power of the capitalist class and enormous weakness of the working class explains why health care reform failed again.[34]

—Vicente Navarro, M.D., professor of public policy,
sociology and policy studies at the Johns Hopkins University
and editor of the *International Journal of Health Services.*

SOME LESSONS FROM THESE REFORM FAILURES

Among the many lessons from these five failures over a century, these are some that are especially striking:

1. Political compromises have led reform proposals to stray from experience, and health policy principles have become too complex, unwieldy, confusing, bureaucratic and ultimately unworkable.
2. We have long had a class and power problem in this country that we tend to deny or accept, but which allows corporate power and money to dominate the media and political process at the expense of popular will and the public interest.
3. This story of recurrent failures of health care reform carries a theme of American exceptionalism throughout—e.g. we can design our own solutions, our problems in the U.S. are unique, and we don't need to look at other countries' experience. As a result, our health care "system", compared to

most other advanced countries, is exceptionally expensive, poor in access, and worse in outcomes.

4. Our growing medical-industrial complex serves itself far more than the families of ordinary Americans; the profit motive drives health care services and politics more than most other countries would ever accept. The service ethic has become subverted in the quest for profits by insurers, hospital systems, the drug industry and related industries as health care plays to corporate shareholders and Wall Street investors more than to patients.

5. Health care is far too important to not get it right. These repeated failures of health care reform show that we still do not learn from history.

CONCLUDING COMMENT

The above gives us an overview of financing changes over the last century in U.S. health care. In Chapter 5, we will deal with the politics of Obamacare as the sixth major attempt to reform our system, where you will find that most of the themes discussed here have not gone away. Meanwhile, let's move in the next chapter to see how the delivery side of our health care has changed over the last 100 years, all of which bears on the continuing challenges of how best to reform health care in the public interest.

References

1. Burrow, JG. AMA: *Voice of American Medicine*. Baltimore. Johns Hopkins Press, 1963: 144.
2. Starr, P. *The Social Transformation of American Medicine*. New York. Basic Books, 1982: 252-3.
3. Ibid #1: 144-5.
4. Ibid # 2: 237.

5. Cunningham, RC III & Cunningham, RM Jr. *The Blues: A History of the Blue Cross and Blue Shield System*. DeKalb, IL, The Northern Illinois University Press, 1997: 35-6.

6. Ibid # 2: 249-50.

7. Rimlinger, GV. *Welfare Policy and Industrialization in Europe, America and Russia*. New York. Wiley, 1971, 110-12.

8. Gilbert, BB, *British Social Policy, 1914-39*. London. Batsford, 1970, 15.

9. Palmer, KS. A Brief History: Universal Health Care Efforts in the U.S. Presentation at the Annual Meeting of Physicians for a National Health Program. San Francisco, CA, Spring 1999.

10. Ibid # 5: 8-9.

11. Committee on the Costs of Medical Care (CCMC). Medical Care for the American People: The Final Report. Chicago. University of Chicago Press, 1932: 7, 41.

12. Campion, FD. *The AMA and U.S. Health Policy Since 1940*. Chicago. Chicago Review Press, 1984: 117.

13. Rothman, DJ. The public presentation of Blue Cross, 1935-1965, *J. Health Polit Policy Law* 16 (4): 671-93.

14. A National Health Program: Report of the Technical Committee on Medical Care. In: *Interdepartmental Committee to Coordinate Health and Welfare Activities, Proceedings of the National Health Conference*, July 18-20, 1938. Washington DC: U.S. Government Printing Office, 1938: 29-63.

15. Somers, AR, Somers, HM. *Health and Health Care: Policies in Perspective*. Germantown, MD. Aspen Systems Corp, 1977: 179-80.

16. A National Health Program: Message from the president. *Soc Secur Bulletin*. 1945: 8 (12).

17. Ibid # 15.

18. Poen, M. *Harry S Truman versus the Medical Lobby: The Genesis of Medicare*. Columbia. University of Missouri Press, 1979: 85-86.

19. Davies, LE. Warren sworn in, asks party peace. *New York Times* 96:21, January 7, 1947.

20. GOP group opposes Warren health plan. *New York Times* 96:2, January 8, 1947.

21. Peterson, MA. Political influence in the 1990s: From iron triangles to policy networks. *Journal Health Pol Policy Law.* 1993:18(2): 395-448.

22. Michelman, F. Forward. On protecting the poor through the Fourteenth Amendment. The Supreme Court. 1968 term. *Harv L Rev.* 1969: 83:7.

23. Kuttner, R. *Everything for Sale: The Virtues and Limits of Markets*. Chicago. University of Chicago Press, 1997: 114.

24. *New York Times*, February 19, 1971.

25. Ibid # 2: 405.

26. McNerney, WJ. C Rufus Rorem Award Lecture. Big question for the Blues: Where to go from here? *Inquiry* 1996, 33 (2): 110-117.

27. Teach, RL. Health Care Reform: Changes and Challenges. Reform tele-conference draws 4,000. *Medical Group Management Update,* 1993; (November): 1, 4.
28. Gordon, C. *The Clinton Health Care Plan: Dead on Arrival.* Westfield, NJ. Open Magazine Pamphlet Series, 1995.
29. Andrews, C. Profit Fever: *The Drive to Corporatize Health Care and How to Stop It.* Monroe, ME. Common Courage Press, 1995: 49-58.
30. Brundin, J. How the U.S press covers the Canadian health care system. *Int J Health Services* 1993, 23 (2): 275-277.
31. Health Care Notes. *The Texas Observer,* December 24, 1993: 22.
32. Will, GF. Coming next: Clinton's year one. *Newsweek,* January 24, 1994; 123 (4).
33. Ibid # 28.
34. Navarro, V. Why Congress did not enact health care reform. *J Health Polit Policy Law*: 1995, 20: 196-199.

CHAPTER 2

CHANGING LANDSCAPE
OF THE DELIVERY SYSTEM

As one-sixth of the entire economy of the United States, our health care system is a massive subject that is difficult to describe and understand. But looking at just two key elements—how it is financed (as we just discussed in the last chapter) and how it is delivered—tells us much of what we need to know. In each case, by tracing how both those parts have come to be over the last century gives us even more understanding of where we are today and where we have to go to address system problems.

As with financing, the delivery side has seen enormous changes. So here, let's ask three basic questions—what, where and how have health care services been delivered in this country, and what have been the major trends over the last century?

DAWN OF THE 20TH CENTURY

Medical care was rudimentary, with hardly an organized system and with minimal quality standards. As in Europe at the time, physicians were being trained by a preceptorship system. Many of our 151 medical schools had no attachment to hospitals and were diploma mills run by five or six local physicians with the support of student fees. Standards for teaching and licensing were lax.[1]

Most physicians were general practitioners in solo office practice at the turn of the century. With no vaccines or antibiotics yet available, infectious diseases were rampant and took a high toll. Average longevity at birth was 48 years for males and 51 years for females.[2]

The scientific revolution soon brought big changes to medical education as many medical schools shifted to universities. Harvard and Johns Hopkins were early leaders in this transition. The AMA established its Council on Medical Education in 1904, for the first time requiring a four-year course of medical studies followed by a one-year internship. The AMA went further to ask the Carnegie Foundation to conduct a rigorous evaluation of U.S. medical schools. Having just finished a critical study of U.S. higher education, Dr. Abraham Flexner was selected to undertake this task. The resulting Flexner Report of 1910 concluded that too many poorly trained physicians were being produced, that there were too many proprietary medical schools with poor standards, and that hospitals with education controls were necessary for medical schools to improve.[3]

The Flexner Report led to great improvements in medical education. Many proprietary medical schools were forced to close as hospitals became actively involved in teaching programs. Hospitals grew after World War I, limited group practice was just starting, some physicians were starting to specialize, but 80 percent were still in general practice in 1930.

THE GREAT DEPRESSION

Starting in 1929 and extending through the 1930s, the Great Depression had a major impact on the delivery of medical care (not yet called health care!) throughout the country. Much of the population lacked the means to pay for care or insurance. Two big changes emerged from this crisis as revenue to hospitals and professionals dropped sharply—the start of direct federal involvement in health care and the growth of a not-for-profit insurance industry.[4]

As part of FDR's New Deal, federal funds were allocated to local health departments for maternal and child health services. The Committee on the Costs of Medical Care (CCMC), mentioned in the last chapter, made these important recommendations (which remain elusive today some 80 years later):

- *Basic public health services should be extended so they will be available to the entire population according to its needs.*

- *The costs of medical care should be placed on a group pay ment basis through the use of insurance or taxation or both.*[5]

Private insurers began offering insurance plans on a not-for-profit basis, providing coverage at discounted rates for hospitals and physicians, in order to help people afford care with minimal out-of-pocket costs and keep hospitals open.[6] Medical underwriting (the process used by health insurers to calculate higher premiums to be charged to individual or group applicants at higher risk for illness), so prevalent today, was considered unethical at the time.

WORLD WAR II

The years during and after World War II saw changes that transformed how health care was delivered in this country. Scientific knowledge expanded greatly, specialization accelerated even as the nation faced a shortage of primary care physicians, groups were starting to replace solo practice, hospitals became the center of a system that was becoming regionalized, and nurses were shifting from private duty to hospital nursing. Voluntary private health insurance was growing rapidly, especially for the employed and their dependents.

THE GREAT SOCIETY: MEDICARE AND MEDICAID

Medicare was enacted with bipartisan support in 1965 at a time when there was widespread concern how the nation's elderly could get and afford medical care. Only about one-half of people 65 years of age and older had any health insurance; those that did found their coverage expensive and meager, with hospital coverage paying for only one-quarter of expenses.[7] Blue Cross was still not-for-profit, but one of its spokesmen admitted that "Insuring everyone over 65 is a losing business that must be subsidized."[8]

Medicare was designed as a social insurance program with universal coverage of a comprehensive set of benefits defined by law without regard to health conditions or income level. Now 49 years old, it has served as a solid rock of coverage for seniors and provided reliable reimbursement to hospitals, physicians and others on the delivery side of health care. Though labeled an entitlement program by critics on the right, it is no such thing. Its benefits are an earned right since beneficiaries have paid into the program through mandatory contributions over the years from individuals and/or employers.[9]

In sharp contrast to the troubled rollout of Obamacare, Medicare was smoothly implemented as universal coverage for a sizable part of the population over a six-month period with a comparatively primitive information system of file cards. Despite today's advances in information technology, such a smooth transition was out of reach today with Obamacare, as it would also have been with the Clinton Health Plan. The reason—both are byzantine in their complexity compared to the simplicity of Medicare in one large risk pool defined only by age.

Medicare was never intended to cover all of the costs of seniors' health care. There was no coverage for prescription drugs, long-term care and some other services. As a result, a large market for supplementary private insurance soon developed. Three of four Medicare beneficiaries carried some kind of supplemental insurance by 1984, generally covering the deductible and coinsurance payments for hospitalization and a 20 percent copayment for physician services.[10]

As we saw in the last chapter, Medicaid, also enacted in 1965, is a partnership between the federal government and the states, but hardly a stable rock of coverage. It is administered by the states, with partial federal funding, and is subject to the vagaries of politics at national and state levels. While it has been helpful for many low-income people, its coverage and eligibility vary widely from one state to another.

CORPORATIZED HEALTH CARE
AND THE MEDICAL-INDUSTRIAL COMPLEX

With new sources of revenue available through Medicare and Medicaid, the delivery side of U.S. health care took off. Several main trends came together—deregulation of markets, expansion of hospitals and other facilities, surplus of specialist physicians (except in primary care), the commodification of health care, growing dominance of hospitals and insurers in a corporate world, and the arrival of managed care. Together, they created a new medical-industrial complex, as first described in 1980 by Dr. Arnold Relman, former editor of *The New England Journal of Medicine.*[11]

The earlier structure of medical practice as a cottage industry, revolving around physicians in solo or small group practice, was long gone. These observations illustrate this transformation:

The intersection in the 1980s and 1990s of a plentiful supply of physicians, the introduction of an underwriting system based on prepayment and shared risk, and the development of large corporations for health care is bringing about a fundamental restructuring of the health services system and a transformation of the practice of medicine.[12]

—Alvin Tarlov, M.D., then president of the Kaiser Family Foundation and chairman of the Council on Graduate Medical Education

Health is industrialized and commercialized in a fashion that enhances many people's dissatisfaction with their health. Advertisers, manufacturers, advocacy groups, and proprietary health care corporations promote the myth that good health can be purchased; they market products and services that purport to deliver the consumer into the promised land of wellness. A giant medical-industrial complex has arisen composed initially of for-profit health care corporations such as free-standing ambulatory surgery centers, free-standing diagnostic laboratories, home health care services, and of course proprietary hospitals.[13]

—Arthur Barsky, professor of psychiatry at Harvard Medical School

Professional power is eroding in two ways, at least. One is through intense competition. Another is through the transfer of power and control from the physician to managers. To some extent, that was inevitable because physicians (with some exceptions) were not willing to step up to the plate and try to deal with the problems of exploding costs and managing the delivery of reasonably good quality care.[14]

—Victor Fuchs, professor emeritus of economics and health
research and policy at Stanford University

The shift away from a physician-centered health care system is well illustrated by Figure 2.1, showing the rapid growth of administrators and managers in the U.S. during these years.[15]

FIGURE 2.1

Growth of Physicians and Administrators 1970-2013

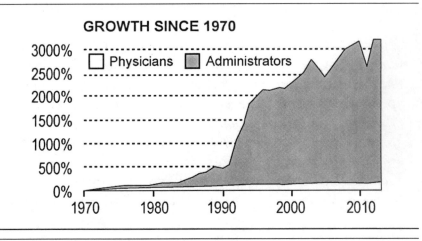

Reprinted with permission from Woolhandler, S, Himmelstein, DU. The National Health Program Slide-Show Guide, Center for National Health Program Studies, Cambridge, MA, 2014.

Managed care brought with it new problems in the late 1980s and 1990s. As a market response to cost containment based on a primary care gatekeeper role as a means to limit referrals, hospitalizations and laboratory tests, it grew rapidly in the form of health maintenance organizations (HMOs) marketed by many new investor-owned for-profit companies. Its business model for maximizing profits trumped service. By the end of the 1990s, many managed care organizations and their HMOs had been discredited for a wide range of deceptive practices, including false advertising[16], under-treatment and denial of services[17], disenrollment of sick enrollees[18], gag rules on physicians[19], hiding performance data[20], and outright fraud.[21] A public and political backlash ensued, so that by 1997 more than 1,000 bills had been introduced into state legislatures in an effort to counter the abuses of the managed care industry.[22]

Under managed care HMO plans, primary care physicians were paid on a capitation basis i.e. so much over a year for caring for so many "covered lives", without regard to how much care those patients required. The incentive was therefore to expand the list of one's patients and shorten their visits. This had a detrimental impact on the doctor-patient relationship, posing a threat to continuity and quality of care.[23] Dr. Kenneth Ludmerer gives us this insight:

Perhaps the most extraordinary development in medical practice during the age of managed care was that time, in the name of efficiency, was being squeezed out of the doctor-patient relationship. Managed care organizations, with their insistence on maximizing "throughput," were forcing physicians to churn through patients in assembly-line fashion at ever-accelerating rates of speed. . . In 1997, doctors on average spent eight minutes talking to each patient, less than half as much time as a decade before.[24]

Table 2.1 compares typical workdays of primary care physicians over the 30-year period from 1980 to 2010. [25, 26]

TABLE 2.1

Comparing the Workday of a Primary Care Physician Now and 30 Years Ago

CRITERION	THEN	NOW
Workday hours	6 or 7 A.M. to 5 or 6 P.M., more if needed at hospital later in day	8 or 9 A.M. to 5 or 6 P.M., more if accessing electronic medical record systems off-site
Chief workday disturbances	Hospital admission or emerging issue with hospital patient	Insurance-related issues (e.g., pre-authorizations) and doing patient call-backs
Variety of work settings	Hospital, office, irregular out-of-office networking opportunities with peers (meetings, etc.)	Office only, few out-of-office networking opportunities with peers
Call schedules	Frequent, daily or every few days	Infrequent, every few days, weeks, or weekends
Oversight of work	Little external oversight of professional standards maintained by PCP individually	Oversight through performance monitoring, and use of standardized clinical guidelines that structure PCP work in many areas
Type of work performed in office	Mostly cognitive medicine, some procedures, some insurance-related patient advocacy work, some coordination of specialist care	Almost all cognitive medicine, regular and increasing insurance-related patient advocacy work, high degree of coordination of specialist care; heavy chronic disease and behavioral health management
Patient expectations	Lower, accepting of delays and going back for information	Higher, expect quicker-turnarounds
Types of patients	Fewer elderly, older chronic-disease populations	More elderly, large chronic-disease populations large at-risk populations, including youth and adolescents
Fiscal reality	Take time with patients, try and do as many things as provider competence and patient needs allow, including procedures—get paid for them; being jack-of all-trades is key strategic goal of provider-keep patient from specialist if you can manage it	Every patient seen quickly is add-itional revenue earned; limiting time with patients key strategic goal of provider-know when it's time to refer patient to specialist, even if you think you can manage it, and refer quickly

Source: Hoff, T. *Practice Under Pressure: Primary Care Physicians and their Medicine in the Twenty First Century*. New Brunswick, NJ, Rutgers University Press, 2010, pp 42-43.

The gatekeeper role was controversial from the start. It put the primary care physician in a difficult bind, bringing a potential conflict of interest into the physician-patient relationship. Dr. Gayle Stephens, a leader in family medicine and former dean of the medical school at the University of Alabama in Huntsville, had this to say about the issue:

> *My experience with contracted gatekeeping is that it is an untenable and hopelessly conflicted role that undermines the volunteerism and earned trust which lies at the heart of the family physician's effectiveness. By introducing elements of compulsion and control into the physician-patient relationship, gatekeeping transforms an intimate, covenantal relationship into a hard-edged contract between strangers—a bad exchange under any circumstances.* [27]

EARLY YEARS OF THE 21ST CENTURY

Spurred on by deregulation and market exuberance launched by the election of President Ronald Reagan in 1980, health care markets have been thriving for the last 30-plus years. This boom has spread through many health-related industries, delighting investors and traders on Wall Street.

But all this has just led to increasing prices and costs of health care and insurance, expanding populations of the uninsured and underinsured, and increasing waste and bureaucracy (mostly in the private sector) that have not given us improved health outcomes. Health care spending has continued its upward climb, well above the cost of living and the ability of ordinary Americans to afford.

These are some of the major trends in recent years:

- Increasing consolidation of the hospital industry, mostly for-profit, with expansion into affiliated ambulatory settings.
- Shift from self-employment of physicians to employment by hospitals and even insurance companies, resulting in less clinical autonomy.

- Emergence of hospitalists, thereby separating inpatient care from outpatient care.
- Increasing corporate monopolies ranging from hospitals to nursing homes and the drug industry.
- Shorter hospital stays and more emphasis on outpatient treatment and home care.
- Growing primary care physician shortage, with increasing fragmentation of care among specialists.
- Rapid adoption of new technologies, even without demonstrated improvements in efficacy or cost-effectiveness.
- Wider use of electronic medical record systems that increase, not decrease physicians' workload, and often don't communicate with each other.
- Return of managed care, despite the discrediting experience of the 1990s.

Private hospital systems and insurers are in the driver's seat in seeking to exploit the public and private purse in expanding markets with few cost or price controls. Large hospital systems have been buying up physician group practices for years as they compete for market share with rival systems. Insurers try to expand their markets by contractual discounted arrangements with physicians, in some cases even employing physicians directly.

Therefore free-wheeling private markets are controlling our so-called health care system, even when our taxpayer dollars are supporting some 60 percent of the system in one way or another. That's hardly news to many of us, but we will see in the next chapter how much collusion has become the norm between a weakened government and the private sector.

References

1. Kaufman, M. American medical education. In: Numbers, RL (ed) *The Education of American Physicians. Historical Essays.* Berkeley, University of California Press, January 1980: 7-28.
2. United States Bureau of the Census. *Historical Statistics of the United States,*

Colonial Times to 1970. Part I. Washington, DC: U.S. Dept. of Commerce, Bureau of the Census, Government Printing Office, 1975: 56.

3. Flexner, A. *Medical Education in the United States and Canada: A Report to the Carnegie Foundation for the Advancement of Teaching.* New York, 1910.

4. Geyman, JP. *Health Care in America: Can Our Ailing System Be Healed?* Boston. Butterworth Heinemann, 2002: 5.

5. Falk, IS. Some lessons from the fifty years since the COMC Final Report, 1932. *J Public Health Policy,* 1983, 4 (2): 139.

6. McNerney, W. C. Rufus Rorem award lecture, Big question for the Blues: Where to go from here? *Inquiry* 1996 (Summer) 33: 110-117.

7. Blumenthal, D, et al. *Renewing the Promise: Medicare & Its Reform.* New York, Oxford University Press, 1988.

8. U.S. Congress. House of Representatives, Committee on Ways and Means, *Medical Care for the Aged,* material submitted for the public record of the hearings on H.R. 3920, Washington, D.C., 1964.

9. *Study Panel on Medicare's Larger Social Role,* Final Report. Washington, D.C. National Academy of Social Insurance, 1999, 31-35.

10. Rice, T. An Economic Assessment of Health Care Coverage for the Elderly. *Milbank Quarterly* 65: 491, 1987.

11. Relman, A. The new medical-industrial complex. *N Engl J Med* 1980: 303: 963-970.

12. Tarlov, AR. Shattuck Lecture—The increasing supply of physicians, the changing structure of the health services system, and the future of medicine. *N Engl J Med* 1993: 308: 1235-1244.

13. Barsky, AJ. The paradox of health. *N Engl J Med* 1988: 318: 414-418.

14. Iglehart, JK. Physicians as agents of social control: The thoughts of Victor Fuchs. *Health Aff (Millwood).* 1998: 17 (1): 91.

15. Woolhandler, S, Himmelstein, DU. The deteriorating administrative efficiency of the U.S. health care system. *N Engl J Med 1991:* 324 (18): 1253-1258.

16. Hellander, I. Quality of care lower in for-profit HMOs than in non-profits. PNHP news release, July 12, 1999.

17. Court, J, Smith, F. *Making a Killing: HMOs and the Threat to Your Health.* Monroe, ME. Common Courage Press, 1999.

18. Morgan, RO et al. The Medicare-HMO revolving door—the healthy go in and the sick go out. *N Engl J Med* 1997: 337: 169-175.

19. Brody, H. Gag rules and trade secrets in managed care contracts. *Arch Intern Med* 1997: 157: 2037-2043.

20. McCormick, D et al. Relationship between low quality-of-care scores and HMO's subsequent disclosure of quality-of-care scores. *JAMA* 2002: 288: 1484.

21. Sparrow, MK. *License to Steal: How Fraud Bleeds America's Health Care System.* Boulder, CO. Westview Press: 2000: 71: 106-107.

22. Mechanic, D. Managed care as a target of distrust. *JAMA* 1997: 277: 1810-1811.

23. Goldberg, RM. What's happened to the healing process? *Wall Street Journal,* June 18, 1997: A22.

24. Ludmerer, KM. Time to Heal: American Medical Education from the Turn of the Century to the Era of Managed Care. New York. Oxford University Press, 1999, p 384.

25. Hoff, T. *Practice Under Pressure*: *Primary Care Physicians and Their Medicine in the Twenty-First Century*. New Brunswick, NJ. Rutgers University Press, 2010, 42-43.
26. Geyman, JP. *Breaking Point: How the Primary Care Crisis Endangers the Lives of Americans*. Friday Harbor, WA. Copernicus Healthcare, 2011: 13.
27. Stephens, GG. Can the family physician avoid a conflict of interest in the gatekeeper role? An opposing view. *J Fam Pract* 1989: 28 (6): 701-704.

CHAPTER 3

PRIVATIZATION AND THE RISE
OF CORPORATE HEALTH CARE

The rise of a corporate ethos in medical care is already one of the most significant consequences of the changing structure of medical care. It permeates voluntary hospitals, government agencies, and academic thought as well as profit-making medical care organizations. Those who talked about "health care planning" in the 1970s now talk about "health care marketing." Everywhere one sees the growth of a kind of marketing mentality in health care. And, indeed, business school graduates are displacing graduates of public health schools, hospital administrators, and even doctors in the top echelons of medical care organizations. The organizational culture of medicine used to be dominated by the ideals of professionalism and volunteerism, which softened the underlying acquisitive activity. The restraint exercised by those ideals now grows weaker. The "health center" of one era is the "profit center" of the next.[1]

—Paul Starr, professor of sociology
at Princeton University and author of
The Social Transformation of American Medicine

Paul Starr made this observation in 1982 about a market-based transformation of U.S. health care. Those trends have become even more dominant and entrenched in the years since, posing real challenges to health care reform. The intertwined trends of privatization and rising corporate dominance in health care have led to corporate vested interests that are coming close to determining health policy with little public governance or accountability.

In this chapter, we will try to bring some historical perspective to this transformation of U.S. health care, with these three objectives: (1) to trace the growth of privatization and corporate transformation across various parts of the delivery system; (2) to examine the claims vs. the realities of privatized health care; and (3) to compare the privatized model with a public utility model of health care.

THE INCREASING PRIVATIZATION
OF HEALTH CARE

Privatization has been the byword and a driving force throughout our economy, particularly over the last three decades, ranging from finance, insurance and real estate (FIRE), prisons, water and the military to schools, information management, and health care. It is based on the unproven assertion that private is better than public programs, that privatizing brings us more efficiencies and better value.

Privatization in health care involves both the private sector and public programs. Sketching the growth of for-profit ownership of different parts of the delivery system since the 1970s gives us a sense of the corporate transformation of medicine and health care.

Hospitals

The traditional freestanding general hospital, serving its own community and governed by its own board, administrators, and medical staff, has almost become a relic of history. For-profit hospital chains emerged in 1968 and grew faster in the 1970s than the computer industry. Some of the chains, such as the Hospital Corporation of America (HCA) even became multi-national corporations with hospitals in many other countries. As Paul Starr has pointed out: "The rise of the for-profit chains has, for the first time, introduced managerial capitalism into American medicine on a large scale."[2]

The two largest hospital chains, HCA (which became Columbia/HCA in 1994) and Tenet Healthcare Corporation (former-ly National Medical Enterprises) are the giants among hospital chains. Each has a long history of aggressive, predatory, even fraudulent business practices. As an example, by 2002 Columbia/ HCA had accumulated a total of $1.7 billion in civil fines and criminal penalties in settlements with the Justice Department.[3] Its fraudulent activities included falsification of patient records, billing for services that were not provided, devious accounting practices, and kickbacks to physicians for patient referrals to their hospitals.[4]

The growth of hospital chains was not limited to acute care hospitals. Founded in 1984, HealthSouth soon became the largest investor-owned chain of rehabilitation hospitals with some 1,800 facilities in all 50 states and abroad. Its flamboyant founder, Rich-ard Scrushy, a former physical therapist, soon ran into trouble with the Justice Department over many fraudulent practices. As one example, he was accused of adding at least $1.4 billion to earnings between 1999 and 2003 and inflating assets by $800 mil-lion in order to lure investors.[5]

Investor-owned for-profit psychiatric hospitals joined the initial rush to corporate chains in the 1970s. They were increas-ing by more than 30 percent a year between 1978 and 1983.[6] But that trend later slowed with cutbacks in mental health coverage by private insurers as psychiatric hospitals became more dependent on Medicare and Medicaid.

Nursing Homes

Until 1970 most nursing homes were small, individually owned facilities tied to their communities. They soon were also caught up by investor-owned chains, which initially thrived on Medicare and Medicaid reimbursement policies that covered operating costs as well as some profit factor. By 1984, the three largest chains—Beverly Enterprises, Hillhaven (subsidiary of Na-tional Medical Enterprises), and ARA Living Centers—operated some 1,500 nursing homes across the country with six times as many beds as not-for-profit nursing homes.[7] Here again, in their quest for profits, nursing home chains were soon found to cut the number of nurses and other staff and fall short of federal standards. In 1997, one-quarter of nursing homes in the country had deficiencies that had either caused actual harm to patients or put them at risk for death or serious injury.[8]

Home Health Care

For-profit, or proprietary home health agencies were banned from Medicare until 1980. But they have grown rapidly since then and now account for a majority of agencies that provide these services. Although Medicare has attempted to upgrade care through a quality monitoring program, recent studies have shown their costs to be higher and quality lower when compared to not-for-profit agencies, belying the claim that for-profits provide better care more efficiently.[9]

Dialysis Centers

German-based Frensenius Medial Care AG acquired National Medical Care (NMC) in 1996, forming Frensenius Medical Care North America (FMCNA). With that acquisition it became the dominant provider of dialysis services with more than 1,000 dialysis clinics across the U.S.[10]

PRIVATIZED HEALTH CARE:
CLAIMS VS. REALITY

Over the last three decades we have heard a continuing drumbeat by proponents of market-based health care that the privatized approach brings us greater efficiency, more choice and value, while also lowering costs through increased competition. That assertion has been made so often as to become a meme, uncritically assumed to be true by many people.

The track record, however, across various parts of the health care industry, is precisely and consistently the opposite—higher costs, restricted choice, less value, and worse quality of care. The only area that privatized care demonstrates new efficiencies is in making money for corporate owners and shareholders. Based on 14 studies from 1999 to 2002, Table 3.1 compares investor-owned care with not-for-profit care in five parts of the health care system.[11]

TABLE 3.1

INVESTOR-OWNED CARE: COMPARATIVE EXAMPLES VS. NOT-FOR-PROFIT CARE

Hospitals	Costs 3-13% higher, with higher overhead, fewer nurses and death rates 6% to 7% higher.
HMOs	Higher overhead (25% to 35% for some of the largest HMOs), worse scores on 14 of 14 quality indicators reported to the National Committee for Quality Assurance.
Dialysis Centers	Death rates 30% higher, with 20% less use of transplants.
Nursing Homes	Lower staffing levels and worse quality of care; 30% committed violations which caused death or life-threatening harm to patients.
Mental Health Centers	Medicare expelled 80 programs after investigations and found that 91% of claims were fraudulent; for-profit behavioral health imposes restrictive barriers and limits to care (eg, premature discharge from hospitals without adequate outpatient care).

Source: Geyman, J.P. *The Corporate Transformation of Health Care: Can the Public Interest Still Be Served?* New York. Springer Publishing Company, 2004, p 228.

When we turn our attention to privatized programs of the public sector—Medicare and Medicaid—the story is much the same: the drive for profits reduces access, choice, and quality of care, while *raising* costs. The history of Medicare is especially interesting. It gained bipartisan support and passage by Congress in 1965 as a "three-layer cake:" Medicare Part A (universal hospitalization coverage for the elderly), Medicare Part B (voluntary, supplemental physician coverage for the elderly), and Medicaid (an expansion of the Kerr-Mills federal-state program for indigent health care). In what became known as "the corporate compromise of 1965," private insurers gained expanded markets of the elderly and poor while being relieved of their worst health risks. Hospitals could anticipate many future years of generous reimbursement for a previously disadvantaged population. The AMA successfully lobbied for a liberal reimbursement system based on a "usual, customary and reasonable" (UCR) reimbursement system.

So from the outset, the federal government was contracting out day-to-day administration of the program to private providers and intermediaries, including claims processing, provider reimbursement, and auditing. With Medicare, private providers and corporations gained new, subsidized markets for expanded populations with higher than normal prevalence of illness. (Fast forward to the 2010 Affordable Care Act: do you see any patterns here?!)

As described in my 2006 book, *Shredding the Social Contract: The Privatization of Medicare,* there were many later (successful) attempts to further privatize Medicare, each based on the unproven premise that the private, competitive marketplace would provide more efficiency, cost savings, value and choice than any government program.[12]

When managed care came along with its promise to save money, payment rates for Medicare HMOs were first set at 95 percent of what traditional Medicare would spend for fee-for-service care in beneficiaries' county of residence. HMOs would not have to share profits with Medicare, and could waive co-insurance and deductibles and offer additional benefits not covered by Medicare.[13]

Such low payments never satisfied the Medicare HMOs, which have successfully lobbied for, and received, much higher overpayments (as much as 20 percent higher), permitted by the government in order to keep them with the program. A recent study of Medicare overpayments to private Medicare plans found that the government made a total of $282.6 *billion* in overpayments between 1985 and 2012. Private plans have been gaming the reimbursement system by selectively enrolling healthier seniors; attempts by the government to risk-adjust payments have failed. The researchers concluded that "Risk adjustment does not work in for-profit private Medicare plans, which have a financial incentive, the data, and the ingenuity to game whatever system Medicare devises."[14]

As for comparisons of Medicare coverage and private Medicare plans, traditional Medicare has been rated more highly than private employer-sponsored insurance consistently over many years. Figure 3.1 shows these differences by five criteria based on a 2001 study by the Commonwealth Fund.[15]

FIGURE 3.1

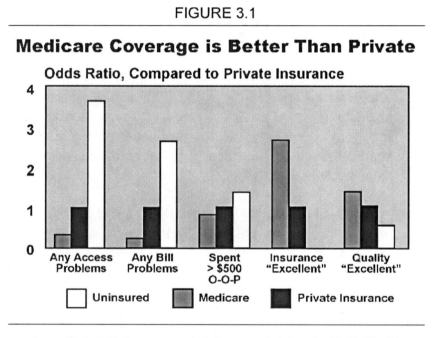

Medicare Coverage is Better Than Private

Odds Ratio, Compared to Private Insurance

Source: Davis, K. Medicare versus private insurance: rhetoric and reality. *Health Affairs Web Exclusive*, Oct. 9, 2002, W311-23
Reprinted with permission from *Health Affairs*

We find the same pattern with privatized Medicaid. Eligibility and coverage vary widely from one state to another, and privatized Medicaid plans also seek to game the reimbursement system to maximize revenue. And as we have seen so clearly in recent years, many governors want to restrict Medicaid, even to the point of refusing 100 percent federal funding for the first two years of Medicaid expansion under the Affordable Care Act.

These examples suggest how little confidence we should have that privatized Medicaid plans will act responsibly:

- A 2003 report found that Medicaid HMOs in New Jersey were tracking down low-income families without telephones, enrolling them, then rejecting 17 to 30 percent of their claims for hospital care.[16]
- In Massachusetts, a 2001 study was done of almost 400,000 Medicaid recipients involved in a joint venture with two of the country's largest for-profit behavioral health companies. These companies took in millions of dollars (without accountability) even as their systems of care collapsed, leaving many covered children stranded unnecessarily in locked wards of psychiatric hospitals without arrangements for outpatient follow-up.[17]

PRIVATIZATION VS. A PUBLIC UTILITY MODEL OF CARE

As you can see from the foregoing, we have evolved a hybrid system over the years since the "corporate compromise of 1965" whereby, even in public programs like Medicare, the government subsidizes the private sector to profiteer at the expense of patients and taxpayers. It has long been obvious that we need more oversight by government and more accountability of privatized programs.

We also need to reexamine and question the assumption that private programs are more efficient, save money, and bring more value than government programs. Private markets work in fundamentally different ways than public programs, in ways that also represent ethical statements of a society. Alan Williams, an English health economist, has conceptualized these differences as libertarian (private) and egalitarian (public) views as shown in Table 3.2.[18]

Just looking at the provider and supply side, for example, shows marked differences in motivation and priorities that end up creating the most expensive system in the world now beset with

TABLE 3.2

Essential Characteristics of Idealized Health Care Systems Based on Libertarian Views (Private Systems) and Egalitarian Views (Public Systems)

System Element	Private System	Public System
Demand	Individuals are the best judges of their own welfare.	When ill, individuals are frequently imperfect judges of their own welfare.
	Priorities are determined by people's own willingness and ability to pay. The erratic and potentially catastrophic nature of demand is mediated by private insurance.	Priorities are determined by social judgments about need. The erratic and potentially catastrophic nature of demand is made irrelevant by the provision of free services.
	Matters of equity are dealt with elsewhere (e.g.. in the tax and Social Security systems).	Since the distribution of income and wealth is unlikely to be equitable in relation to the need for health care, the system must be insulated from its influence.
Supply	Profit is the proper and most effective way to motivate suppliers to respond to the needs of demanders.	Professional ethics and dedication to public service are the appropriate motivation of suppliers, who should focus on success in curing and caring.
Adjustment	Priorities are determined by people's willingness and ability to pay and by the costs of meeting their wishes at the margin.	Priorities are determined by identifying the greatest-improvements in caring or curing that can be effected at the margin.
Mechanics	Well-informed consumers are able to seek out the most cost-effective form of treatment for themselves.	Well-informed clinicians are able to prescribe the most cost-effective form of treatment for each patient.
	If medical practice is profitable at the price that prevails in the market, more people will go into medicine: hence, supply will be demand responsive. If, conversely, medical practice is unrenumerated, people will leave it, or stop entering it, until the system returns to equilibrium.	If there is demand pressure on some facilities or specialties, resources will be directed toward extending them. Facilities or specialties on which demand pressure is slack will be slimmed down to release resources for other uses.
Success Criteria	Consumers will judge the system by their ability to get somone to do what they demand, when, where, and how they want it done.	The electorate judges the system by the extent to which it improves the health status of the population at large in relation to resources allocated to it.
	Producers will judge the system by how substantial a living they can make through it.	Producers judge the system by its ability to enable them to provide the treatment they believe to be cost-effective.

Source: William A. Priority setting in needs-based system. In: Committee on *Technological Innovatrion in Medicine, Geligns AC (ed.). Technology and Health Care in an Era of Limits, Washington DC: National Academy Press, 1992: 79-95.* Reprinted with permission by the National Academy of Sciences, courtesy of the National Academies Press, Washington D.C.

uncontrollable prices, increasing bureaucracy (especially on the private side), and unsustainable trends.

Medicare gives us a window to examine the track record of a program over almost 50 years in terms of its political history. As we have seen, it was partly privatized from the beginning by delegating administrative responsibility to local and regional private insurers. Later privatized additions include management of the prescription drug benefit and the two private health plans— Medicare + Choice and its successor Medicare Advantage. Our experience with both privatized health plans over 25-some years is well summarized in Table 3.3 in ways that we could have predicted from the start.[19]

It has been disappointing to watch continued efforts over many years by the Republicans to "save Medicare" by further privatization. In 1995, for example, the new Republican majority in Congress, as part of its Contract with America, brought a bill forward that would have shifted Medicare to a program with defined contributions instead of benefits defined by law.[20] Newt Gingrich, as Speaker of the House, declared that this kind of "reform" would "solve the Medicare program" and cause it to "wither on the vine." [21, 22] The longer-term strategy, of course, was to profit from privatized plans that would segment the risk pool of healthier seniors into private plans, leave sicker seniors in traditional Medicare with increasing costs, then cut government spending by "premium support" or voucher plans.

In his 2003 book, *The Political Life of Medicare*, Jonathan Oberlander observed the long-standing political battle over markets versus the government in public policy:

> *Medicare politics is now transparently a battle of ideas about the role of markets and government in public policy. This is, in many respects, the same debate held in the 1950s and 1960s before Medicare's enactment, replete with the same sharp partisan cleavages, high-visibility politics that reach into national elections, a broad scope of conflict, and an engaged public. The new politics of Medicare is an echo of the past.*[23]

Fast forward to today's politics over "entitlement programs." The ongoing battle over Medicare and Medicaid reflects little change in this fundamental, long unresolved question of the role of markets in public programs. Representative Paul Ryan's voucher plan for Medicare would be a defined contribution way of shifting

TABLE 3.3

Comparative Features of Privatized and Public Medicare

PRIVATIZED MEDICARE	ORIGINAL MEDICARE
Experience-rated eligibility	Universal coverage
Managed competition	Social insurance as earned
Defined contribution	Defined benefits
Segmented risk pool	Broad risk pool
Market pricing to risk	Administered prices
More volatile access & benefits	More reliable access & benefits
Increased cost sharing	Less cost sharing
Less accountability	Potential for more accountability
Less choice of provider & hospital	Full choice of provider & hospital
Less well distributed	Well distributed
Less efficiency, higher overhead	More efficiency, lower overhead

Source: Geyman, JP. *Shredding the Social Contract The Privatization of Medicare.* Monroe, ME. Common Courage Press, 2006: p. 206.

more costs of care to seniors, leaving them more vulnerable to the high costs of care in their age group. The Congressional Budget Office (CBO) has already calculated that seniors would pay much more for health care under this "premium support" plan.[23] Meanwhile, as a current example of Republican politics in a red state, Louisiana's Governor Bobby Jindal is overseeing the privatization of nine of the state's ten public hospitals, including Louisiana State University's main teaching hospital and other safety net hospitals. It is expected that more than 5,000 employees will be laid off in the wake of these privatizations.[25, 26] Based on past history of privatized Medicaid programs, we can only anticipate this move to result in decreased access and worse outcomes of care for a large disadvantaged population.

These two observations over this span of history sum up where we have been and are now in U.S. health care:

No other nation expects a private sector, little constrained by public rules on the size and terms of employer contributions, to carry so heavy a burden of coverage, and none asks private insurers to hold the line with providers (including specialists, uncommonly abundant in the United States) on prices outside a framework of public policies that guide the bargaining game. The first of these two grand exceptions largely accounts for the nation's high rates of un- and underinsurance; the latter mainly explains why American health spending is so high by cross-national standards.[27]

—Lawrence D. Brown, professor of health policy and management at Columbia University

U.S. health policies have failed to meet national needs during the past four decades because they have been heavily influenced by the delusion that medical care is essentially a business . . . The current rate of inflation of health care costs is unsustainable, and it is likely that any market-based solutions will fail to address the problem. . . . A real solution to our crisis will not be found until the public, the medical profession and government reject the prevailing delusion that health care is best left to market forces.[28]

—Arnold S. Relman, M.D., former editor of *The New England Journal of Medicine* and author of *A Second Opinion: Rescuing America's Healthcare.*

We have seen how private markets work in health care. Now it is time to turn, in the next chapter, to what this means for values and ethics.

References

1. Starr, P. *The Social Transformation of American Medicine*. New York. Basic Books. 1982: 448.
2. Ibid # 1: 430-431.
3. Associated Press. Hospital chain ends fraud case. *New York Times*, December 19, 2002: C9.
4. Sparrow, MK. *License to Steal: How Fraud Bleeds America's Health Care System*. Boulder, CO. Westview Press, 2000.
5. Norris, F. In U.S. eyes, a fraud particularly bold. *New York Times*, March 20, 2003: C1.
6. Gray, BH. (ed) *For-Profit Enterprise in Health Care*. Washington, D.C. Institute of Medicine, National Academy Press, 1986.
7. Ibid # 6: 32-33.
8. Harrington, C et al. Does investor-ownership of nursing homes compromise the quality of care? *American Journal of Public Health* 2001: 91: 1.
9. Cabin, W, Himmelstein, DU, Siman, ML et al. For-profit Medicare home health agencies' costs appear higher and quality appears lower compared to non-profit agencies. *Health Affairs*, August 2014.
10. Frensenius Medical Care reports third quarter and nine months 2005 results; outlook for 2005 confirmed. www.fmc-na.com. Accessed February 13, 2006.
11. Geyman, JP. *The Corporate Transformation of Health Care: Can the Public Interest Still Be Served?* New York. Springer Publishing Company. 2004: 228.
12. Geyman, JP. *Shredding the Social Contract: The Privatization of Medicare*. Monroe, ME. Common Courage Press, 2006: 52-64.
13. King, KM, Schlesinger, M. (eds) *Final Report of the Study Panel on Medicare and Markets: Lessons from the Past, Looking to the Future*. Washington, D.C. National Academy of Social Insurance, September 2003: 607-608.
14. Hellander, I, Himmelstein, DU, Woolhandler, S. Medicare overpayments to private plans, 1985-2012: shifting seniors to private plans has already cost Medicare $282.6 billion. *Intl J Health Services* 43 (2): 305-319, 2013.
15. Davis, K. Medicare versus private insurance; rhetoric and reality. *Health Aff Web Exclusive*, October 9, 2003: W 311-323.
16. Freudenheim, M. Some concerns thrive on Medicaid patients. *New York Times*, February 19, 2003: C1.
17. Wolfe, SM. Unhealthy partnership: How Massachusetts and its managed care contractor shortchange troubled children. *Public Citizen Health Research Group Letter* 2001: 17 (2): 1.
18. Williams, A. Priority setting in a needs-based system. In: Committee on Technological Innovation in Medicine. Institute of Medicine. Gelijns, AC. (ed) *Technology and Health Care in an Era of Limits*. Washington, D.C. National Academy Press, 1992: 79-95.
19. Ibid # 11: 206.

20. Ibid # 12: 5-16.
21. Hacker, JS. *The Divided Welfare State: The Battle Over Public and Private Social Benefits in the United States*. Cambridge. Cambridge University Press, 2002: 329.
22. Smith, DG. *Entitlement Politics: Medicare and Medicaid 1995-2001*. New York. Aldine de Gruyter, 2002: 71, citing *Congressional Quarterly Almanac*, 1995: 7-13.
23. Oberlander, J. *The Political Life of Medicare*. Chicago. University of Chicago Press, 2003: 196.
24. Congressional Budget Office. Long-term analysis of a budget proposal by Chairman Ryan, April 5, 2011.
25. Bannon, EP. Nine of Louisiana's ten public hospitals to be privatized. World Socialist Web Site, May 30, 2013.
26. Associated Press. Bobby Jindal won't scrap Louisiana hospital privatization model. May 5, 2014.
27. Brown, LD. In Stevens, RA, Rosenberg, CE, Burns, LR. (eds) *History and Health Policy in the United States: Putting the Past Back In*. New Brunswick, NJ. Rutgers University Press, 2006: 46.
28. Relman, AS. The health of nations. *The New Republic*, March 7, 2005.

CHAPTER 4

A SEA CHANGE IN VALUES:
FROM SERVICE TO A BUSINESS "ETHIC"

Few trends could so thoroughly undermine the very foundations of our free society as the acceptance by corporate officials of a social responsibility other than to make as much money for their shareholders as possible.[1]

—Milton Friedman, author of *Capitalism and Freedom* and Nobel laureate in economics

We are not real believers in the free-market mechanism unless we can honestly say that we would be willing to see some patients suffer the consequences if they could not afford an available treatment being provided to wealthier patients. . . . Health care costs are being treated as if they were largely an economic problem, but they are not. To be solved, they will have to be treated as an ethical problem.[2]

—Lester Thurow, Ph.D., economist and former dean of the MIT Sloan School of Management

The above quotes reflect polar opposites in how our health care system should be designed and operated. As we saw from the last chapter, Friedman's approach has proven dominant as health care has been commodified and privatized within a commercial and corporate culture over the last 40 years.

This chapter has three objectives: (1) to trace how a traditional service ethic within today's health care system and the medical profession has been taken over by a business "ethic" to maximize profits; (2) to consider to what extent pushback has taken place in the corporate sector and within the medical profession; and (3) to very briefly summarize some of the consequences of these changes for physicians, patients and families, business, and society.

FROM SERVICE TO A PROFIT-DRIVEN INDUSTRY

The Corporate Takeover of Health Care.

We saw in the last chapter how extensive this corporate take-over of health care has been. Harkening back to the power of the "invisible hand" in the writings of Adam Smith, market proponents keep assuring us that competitive free markets are self-regulating.

But a brief survey of large players across the medical-industrial complex soon belies any claim to self-regulation. Instead, the pursuit of profits by any means shows how unethical practices abound, as these examples illustrate.

Insurers

- Discount health plans are a new product targeting uninsured and underinsured whereby patients pay a monthly or annual fee up front to get a card that is supposed to give access to a network offering reduced charges for physician visits, prescription drugs and other services. State regulators have been cracking down since many of the networks have few providers, discounts can be much less than advertised, and some of the plans are illegitimate.[3]

Hospitals

- Health Management Associates (HMA) is a for-profit hospital chain based in Naples, Florida, with more than 200 facilities. The Justice Department has joined eight separate whistle-blower lawsuits against HMA in six states over its practices pressuring emergency room doctors to admit more patients to the hospital. One target benchmark is to admit at least one-half of patients over age 65, whether they need hospital care or not. Coordinated strategies are used to meet target benchmarks, including colored scorecards in emergency rooms, sophisticated software programs, financial incentives, threats, and even firing of physicians or executives who do not go along with these practices.[4] In late January 2014, Community Health Systems, based in Franklin, Tennessee, completed its acquisition of HMA to become the country's largest for-profit hospital chain.[5]

- HCA, then the largest for-profit hospital chain in the country with 163 hospitals from New Hampshire to California, was bought in 2006 by three private equity firms, including Bain Capital, co-founded by Mitt Romney. It thrived during the Great Recession by billing insurers, Medicare and patients more aggressively than before.[6] This is the same HCA that paid the largest health care fraud settlement in U.S. history—$1.7 billion—in 2003.[7]

Nursing homes

- A 2011 study of the ownership, financing and management strategies of the ten largest for-profit nursing home chains in the U.S. found that: "the chains have used strategies to maximize shareholder and investor value that include increasing Medicare revenues, occupancy rates, and company diversification, developing real estate investment trusts, and creating limited liability companies. These strategies enhance shareholder and investor profits, reduce corporate taxes, and reduce liability risk. There is a need for greater transparency in ownership and financial reporting and for more government oversight of the largest for-profit chains, including those owned by private equity companies."[8]
- In late 2014, Extendicare, one of the largest nursing home chains in the country with about 150 homes in 11 states, agreed to pay $38 million to settle federal charges that it billed inappropriately for physical therapy and provided unnecessary and inadequate care; cutbacks in the numbers of trained

nurses and their emphasis on the business model led to pervasive problems in patient care, including malnutrition, dehydration, and high rates of falls and infections.[9]

Drug industry

- In 2012, the Drug Enforcement Administration (DEA) blocked four pharmacies in Sanford, Florida, including two CVS pharmacies, from selling controlled substances. It turned out that Cardinal Health, the second largest pharmaceutical distributor in the country, had been shipping to these four pharmacies 50 times the volume of oxycodone shipped to the average pharmacy in Florida, and that it had been fined $34 million four years earlier to settle allegations that it had failed to prevent supplies from being diverted.[10]
- Phase IV drug trials, also known as "seeding trials", are typically run by drug companies' *marketing* departments. With no federal human subject protections, these "studies" have no scientific rigor or credibility, and can be dangerous for patients. In a twelve-year seeding trial of Neurontin, a Pfizer seizure drug, 11 patients died during the study and 73 others had serious adverse events, none of which were publicized. It was clear from later litigation documents that this "study" was more marketing than research.[11]
- The drug industry continues to pressure the FDA to accelerate drug reviews and give it more leeway to promote its products while relaxing reporting requirements over safety concerns, in spite of its record of having one-third of approved drugs receiving black-box warning labels or being withdrawn from the market for safety reasons.[12]

Medical devices

- When its all-metal ASR hip replacement was found defective, the DePuy orthopedic division of Johnson & Johnson continued to market it overseas and marketed a closely related implant in this country through a regulatory loophole not requiring evidence of safety and effectiveness. The company finally recalled these devices after failure rates continued to grow both here and abroad, resulting in the filing of some 5,000 lawsuits against the company.[13]

- For-profit dialysis centers have been found to increase their profits by using shorter dialysis periods and reusing manufactured dialyzers that are labeled for single use in just one patient.[14]

Health care fraud

This has become epidemic and is still uncontrolled, intertwined as it is with complex billing practices throughout the system. Professor Malcolm Sparrow, Ph.D., as an experienced detective, former detective chief inspector with the British police service, faculty member at Harvard, and author of the classic book, *License to Steal: How Fraud Bleeds America's Health Care System*, tells us that:

> *[Health care fraud] represents one of the most massive and persistent fiscal control failures in our history. Many who work the system, or feed off it, like it so. For those who profit from it, health care fraud is not seen as a problem, but as an enormously lucrative enterprise, worth defending vigorously.*[15]

Sparrow's book describes how pervasive and embedded fraud is across the entire health care system, and how resistant it has been to control by regulators. This warning shows how difficult it will be to address this problem:

> *It is no longer sensible to disburse public funds, on trust, through electronic systems. The commensurate risks are enormous, and seriously underestimated. . . . Absent some fundamental reassessment of electronic payment systems, we are doomed to continue dealing with serious fraud threats on a case-by-case basis rather than on a structural basis. Happily, each case detected provides some (false)*

assurance because it was, after all, detected. And each successive scandal offers an opportunity for officials to proclaim, once again, their 'zero tolerance' for fraud in vital public programs.[16]

So much for self-regulation by deregulated free markets. As Joseph Stiglitz, Nobel laureate in economics and former chief economist at the World Bank, sums up their track record:

Unlike his followers, Adam Smith was aware of some of the limitations of free markets, and research since then has further clarified why free markets, by themselves, often do not lead to what is best. As I put it in my new book, Making Globalization Work, the reason that the invisible hand often seems invisible is that it is often not there . . . some regulation is required to make markets work.[17]

The Ethical Transformation of Medicine

The medical profession and medical practice had a long tradition of service before it underwent its transformation from a service-oriented cottage industry into big business controlled by investor-owned corporate stakeholders. Its history shows the magnitude of this change.

William Osler (1849-1919), the best-known physician and medical educator in the English-speaking world at the turn of the 20th Century, believed that beneficence should be an integral part of the physician's role:

As the practice of medicine is not a business and can never be one, the education of the heart—the moral side of the man—must keep pace with the education of the head. . . . The profession of medicine is distinguished from all others by its singular beneficence.[18]

Graduates of medical schools in most countries around the world take one or another kind of oath, such as the Hippocratic

Oath and the Physician's Oath. While they vary in details, there is a common theme of beneficence running through them that transcends culture, religion, and historical time.

Despite these traditions emphasizing service, there has been a long-standing tension among physicians between altruistic service to patients and entrepreneurial self-interest. Dr. Edmund Pellegrino, internist and a leading medical ethicist at Georgetown University, identified the dilemma facing the medical profession as a choice between two opposing moral orders, "one based in the primacy of our ethical obligations to the sick, the other to the primacy of self-interest and the marketplace."[19]

Dr. Jonas Salk gives us a good example of the traditional service ethic untarnished by personal gain. With some funding support from the March of Dimes, he developed the first effective polio vaccine in 1955, which soon was in big demand. But neither he nor his sponsor would patent the vaccine. Edward R. Murrow asked him who owned the patent. Salk's answer: "The American people, I guess. Could you patent the sun?"[20]

After reviewing the enormous changes in the health care marketplace in the last chapter, including the growing dominance of investor-owned corporate health care, it is both predictable and understandable that the medical profession has been engulfed by changing incentives in the new marketplace.

In his book, *A Short History of Medical Ethics*, Dr. Albert Jonsen, bioethicist and former chairperson of the University of Washington's Department of Medical History and Ethics, describes the dilemma confronting physicians today in this country:

> *The encounter between patient and physician is no longer a private place. It is a cubicle with open walls, surrounded by a crowd of managers, regulators, financiers, producers and lawyers required to manage the flow of money that makes the encounter possible. All of them can look into the encounter and see opportunities for profit or economy. All would like to have a say in how the encounter goes—from the time consumed by it, to the drugs prescribed in it, to the costing out of each of its elements*[21]

The medical profession must bear part of the responsibility for not standing up for patients and challenging the changes that have made health care so expensive that it is now beyond the reach of so many tens of millions of ordinary Americans. Physicians order almost all of the health services that patients receive. And physicians increasingly have conflicts of interest, including ownership and/or investments in health care facilities where they can increase their profits doubly or triply beyond the services they actually rendered.

In my 2008 book, *The Corrosion of Medicine: Can the Profession Reclaim Its Moral Legacy?*, I described many ways whereby the medical profession has strayed from its noble traditions of the past. Here are just a few examples in recent years that show how pervasive these departures are and how fully they fall into the area of self-interest.[22]

• *Conflicts of interest with the drug industry*

These are widespread within the profession, including acceptance of highly paid roles as "consultants" to drug companies, giving talks more oriented to marketing than unbiased science; accepting "educational grants" with no strings attached and no reports required; and financial involvement with drug companies, without disclosure, as "experts" developing clinical practice guidelines for use of drugs for which guidelines were being written.

In 2003, the drug industry provided about 90 percent of funding for continuing medical education (CME) in the U.S.[23]; in return, drug companies can often help with design of CME programs and selection of speakers, openly acknowledging that they fund only those programs that are most likely to be profitable.[24]

As a result of the Physician Payments Sunshine Act, included as a provision in the ACA, a recent report found $3.5 billion worth of financial ties between physicians and academic medical centers and drug and medical device makers in the last five months of 2013. Most of these payments were made directly to physicians, mostly involving research, including compensation for consultation and speaking fees; $1 billion went to medical providers with ownership stakes in their companies.[25]

• *Conflicts of interest with the medical device industry*

The medical device industry brings to market some 8,000 products each year, most of which are loosely regulated by the FDA. Manufacturers seek out physicians to use and promote their products as a major part of their marketing programs. As one example, Medtronic, the largest medical device manufacturer in the industry, spent at least $50 million in payments to physicians between 2001 and 2003 as part of its marketing program; that included payments of $400,000 a year to one surgeon for a consulting contract requiring just eight days of work.[26]

There are now surgeon-owned implant companies for spinal surgery in 20 states, and they are moving into such other areas as cardiac, hip, and knee surgery. In this way, surgeon owners "double dip" by using devices made by their companies.[27]

• *Specialty hospitals*

Physician-owned specialty hospitals have emerged over the last 25 years in an effort to evade laws that prohibit them from referring their patients to hospitals in which they are invested. But they do just that, most focusing on well-reimbursed procedures in cardiovascular disease, orthopedic surgery, and neurosurgery. Although they claim to offer more efficiency and value for patients, it is obvious that maximizing income is a major driver. Specialty hospitals cherry pick well insured patients, while physician owners can "triple dip" by receiving income from performing a procedure, sharing in a facility profit, and increasing the value of their investment in the business.[28]

• *Ambulatory surgery centers (ASCs)*

There are more than 4,000 ASCs across the country, usually privately owned between hospitals and physicians, sometimes entirely owned by physicians and investors. Conflicts of interest are so widespread that a 2003 *Medical Economics* article described ways in which physician investors might avoid anti-kickback regulations.[29]

- *Imaging centers*

Physician owners of CT and other imaging equipment order two to eight times as many imaging procedures as those who do not own such equipment; this amounts to some $40 billion worth of unnecessary imaging each year.[30]

Taken together, these kinds of changes show how pervasively the medical profession collectively has fallen away from the public interest in serving its own interests. Most of its organizations have been part of this process. The profession has let patients down. Dr. David Lotto, a psychoanalytic historian, says this about the corporate takeover of the soul of medical practice and health care:

There are far too many health professionals among us who are willing to bend, contort, and turn inside out, our traditional professional values. Too many are willing to accommodate to the values of the corporate world where protecting the wealth of those who are paying you becomes a legitimate part of your professional function. Making this kind of accommodation has its rewards: mainly financial security and a comfortable middle-class lifestyle. But like all such Faustian bargains, there is a steep price to pay. The problem is that in order to avoid anxiety and guilt we come to share the moral blind spot of our corporate culture.[31]

ANY PUSHBACK TO STRENGTHEN THE SERVICE ETHIC?

We have seen the relentless envelopment of health care by corporate stakeholders profiting from expanded markets. We cannot expect any pushback from them. But some are sensitive to growing public opinion over their excesses, so make some efforts to burnish their image.

General Electric (GE), as the 12th largest corporation in the world, is a case in point. It has tentacles in health care that range from imaging equipment and information management to robotics. It also has major holdings in the insurance industry, financial services and the media, including ownership of NBC. Concerned about growing anti-corporate public opinion in the wake of negative publicity around the retirement benefits of its former CEO, Jack Welch, it launched a $100 million public relations campaign in 2003 to improve its image, including changing its corporate slogan from "We bring good things to life" to "Imagination at work." The intent was to downplay its enormous scale and promote its spirit of innovation.[32]

All that, of course, was just posturing and trying to change the subject. As one of the behemoth corporate giants across the globe, it is positioned to garner profits around the world without public accountability. William Greider, well-known political journalist and author of *The Soul of Capitalism: Opening Paths to a Moral Economy*, has described its political prowess as a global corporation in these words:

> *Given its girth and skill and other attributes, a politically active corporation like General Electric acts like a modern version of the 'political machine', with some of the same qualities of the old political machines that used to dominate American cities.*[33]

GE's record on health care issues is both predictable and self-serving. In 2002, without disclosure of its conflict of interest, its *NBC News* misrepresented the issues surrounding Oregon's Initiative 23 for single-payer universal coverage.[34] It has opposed any examination of its business practices by *NBC News*.[35] As high costs drive many patients to pay their bills with "medical credit cards," GE charges rates up to 26.99 percent for its CareCredit card.[36]

Many physicians have tried to uphold their traditional principles based on a service ethic, but have found themselves unable to confront the system and swamped by this tidal wave of commercialism. Faced with increasing office overhead and competition from expanding hospital systems, many have no longer been able to afford to remain in independent practice. An increasing number are considering early retirement or leaving medicine altogether.

Many physicians, perhaps most, are honest, hard-working and still place their patients' best interests above their own. There are many excellent examples of professionalism in many parts of the system, especially in rural and underserved areas, and in other safety net programs. But most feel trapped in a system over which they have little or no control.

Some medical organizations have stood up for the service ethic in response to the onslaught of corporate profit-driven change, as illustrated by these groups: Physicians for Social Responsibility (PSR), Physicians for a National Health Program (PNHP), National Medical Association (NMA), American Women's Medical Association (AMWA), American Medical Students Association (AMSA), American Public Health Association (APHA), and the American Society for Bioethics and Humanities, to name a few. A new *Charter on Medical Professionalism* was developed as a joint effort by three internal medicine organizations (American Board of Internal Medicine Foundation, American College of Physicians-American Society of Internal Medicine Foundation, and the European Federation of Internal Medicine) emphasizing three core principles—primacy of patient welfare, patient autonomy, and social justice.[37]

But despite the best efforts of these organizations, they have been swamped by commercialism, with which many physicians have been complicit and profited from. Most medical and specialty organizations have been more concerned with their own self-interest, continuing to support a market-based approach with little regulation. The AMA, with a membership today of less than 20 percent of professionally active U.S. physicians, still plays a reactionary role opposing universal access to health care, as it has since 1917.

Dr. Carl Elliott, physician, philosopher and professor at the Center for Bioethics at the University of Minnesota, describes the current situation this way:

Without actually intending it, we have constructed a medical system in which deception is often not just tolerated but rewarded. A series of social and legislative changes have transformed medicine into a business, yet because of medicine's history as a self-regulating profession, no one is really policing it. On the surface, our medical system looks very similar to the way it looked twenty-five years ago. Dig deeper, though, and you can see the same patterns of misconduct emerging again and again.[38]

CONSEQUENCES OF THIS SEA CHANGE ON ETHICS AND VALUES

As we have seen, the impact of corporate health care has had a profound and deleterious effect on how medicine is practiced today.

These are some of the adverse impacts on physicians:

- Loss of professional sovereignty
- Loss of clinical autonomy
- Increased practice dissatisfaction and burnout
- Increased entrepreneurialism
- New conflicts of interest as employees of employers with whom they disagree on values
- Erosion of public trust

Between 1965 and 1999, numerous national surveys showed the medical profession in this country to decline from one of the most trusted to one of the least trusted social institutions.[39,40]

For patients, this 2003 observation by Emily Friedman, ethicist and health policy analyst, is even more true today in summarizing the plight of so many patients as they try to navigate our so-called system:

The health care system makes patients feel powerless, and it makes many of those who work within it feel exactly the same way. But until we change the infrastructure and the corporate culture of health care, until the fiefdoms and the turfs and the lust for money and the competition and the power positions are broken down, until teamwork replaces individual arrogance and patients replace power mongers as the focus of the system, innocent people will continue to be terrified, humiliated, injured and killed unnecessarily— not because of any individual wrongdoing, but because the system does not and cannot serve them well.[41]

For the business community, except to the extent that corporate health care makes profits, the rest of business falls under an increasing burden of costs. Its long-standing social contract with employees is rapidly falling apart. Employer-sponsored insurance (ESI) continues its decline as more expenses are turned over to workers.

For society, as the health care debate takes center stage over Obamacare and the way forward, health care is a hot and divisive issue that divides Americans and weakens social solidarity. Our fundamental questions are still unanswered, such as "Who is the health care system for?", and "Should health care be a human right or just another commodity available to people based on ability to pay?"

We started this chapter with two polar opposite views, and will end the same way. Whose side are we on in 21st century America?

Do we have an obligation to provide health care for everybody? Where do we draw the line? Is any fast-food restaurant obligated to feed everyone who shows up?[42]

—Richard Scott, co-founder, chairman, CEO and president of Columbia/HCA Healthcare Corporation until he was fired over a $1.7 billion fraud settlement, and now governor of Florida

In the end, money is a cruel god, not worthy of devotion. And this is perhaps the clearest way of saying what is troubling about this elusive but all-important interior

and motivational dimension of the hegemony of money in medicine: the cruelty lies in the way money overpowers all other values and thereby uproots physicians of the deep rewards of recognizing themselves as part of a healing process. Money (and the considerable list of things it can buy) becomes the chief standard against which doctors judge themselves and seek to be judged. But for professionals the only god worthy of solemn devotion is signified in the etymology of 'profession,' viz., an avowal of service beyond self.[43]

—Larry Churchill, Ph.D., well-known bioethicist
at Vanderbilt University

References

1. Friedman, M. Capitalism and Freedom. Chicago. University of Chicago Press, 1967.
2. Thurow, LC. Sounding Board: Learning to say "No." *N Engl J Med* 311 (24): 1571, 1984.
3. Mertens, M. Consumer confusion triggers crackdown by states on discount health plans. *Kaiser Health News*, April 28, 2010.
4. Creswell, J, Abelson, R. Hospital chain said to inflate bills. *New York Times*, January 23, 2014.
5. Kutscher, B. CHS-HMA deal hikes pressure on smaller systems, hospitals. *Modern Healthcare*, January 27, 2014.
6. Creswell, J, Abelson, R. A giant hospital chain is blazing a profit trail. *New York Times*, August 14, 2012.
7. Soeken,DR. *International Whistleblower Archive.* (www.whistleblowing.us)
8. Harrington, C, Hauser, C, Olney, B, Rosenau, PV. Ownership, financing, and management strategies of the ten largest for-profit nursing home chains in the United States. *Intl J Health Services* 41 (4): 725-746, 2011.
9. Thomas, K. Chain to pay $38 million over claims of poor care. *New York Times*, October 10, 2014.
10. Barrett, D, Martin, TW. Pharmacies swept into drug wars. *Wall Street Journal*, February 15, 2012: B1.

11. Krumholtz, SD, Egilman, DS, Ross, JS. Study of Neurontin: titrate to effect, profile of safety (STEPS) trial. *Arch Intern Med* 171 (12): 1100-1107, 2011

12. Frank, C, Himmelstein, DU, Woolhandler, S et al. Era of faster FDA drug approval has also seen increased black-box warnings and market withdrawals. *Health Affairs*, August 2014.

13. Meier, B. Hip implants U.S. rejected sold overseas. *New York Times*, February 12, 2012: A1.

14. Himmelstein, DU, Woolhandler, S, Hellander, I. *Bleeding the Patient: The Consequences of Corporate Health Care*. Monroe, ME. Common Courage Press, 2001.

15. Sparrow, MK. *License to Steal: How Fraud Bleeds America's Health Care System*. Boulder, Co. Westview Press, 2000, p. xvii.

16. Sparrow, MK. An e-ripoff of the U.S. Disbursing public funds electronically sets up the federal government to be victimized by massive fraud. *Los Angeles Times* on line, August 21, 2011.

17. Stiglitz, JE. As quoted in Altman, D. *Managing Globalization*. In Q & Answers with Joseph E. Stiglitz, Columbia University and *The International Herald Tribune*, October 11, 2006.

18. Osler, W. On the Educational Value of the Medical Society. In: Aequanimitas, With Other Addresses to Medical Students, Nurses, and Practitioners of Medicine. 3rd edition. Philadelphia, PA.

19. Pellegrino, ED. The medical profession as a moral community. *Bull N Y Acad Med* 66 (3): 221, 1990.

20. Smith, J. *Patenting the Sun: Polio and the Salk Vaccine*. New York. William Morrow, 1990: 159.

21. Jonsen, A. Opening remarks. Symposium on Commercialism in Medicine. Program in Medicine & Human Values. California Pacific Medical Center, San Francisco: September 2005. *Cambridge Quarterly of Health Care*, spring 2007.

22. Geyman, JP. *The Corrosion of Medicine: Can the Profession Reclaim Its Moral Legacy?*. Monroe, ME. Common Courage Press, 2008: 118-136.

23. ACCME annual report data 2003. Chicago. Accreditation Council for Continuing Medical Education, 2003.

24. The Pharmaceutical Research and Manufacturers of America (PhRMA). HHS OIG compliance program guidance for the pharmaceutical industry: key insights from regulators and compliance experts. In: PhRMA Congress Conference, Spring 2003: June 8-9, 2003. Washington, D.C.

25. Terhune, C, Levey, NN, Poindexter, S. Database shows $3.5 billion in industry ties to doctors, hospitals. *Los Angeles Times*, September 30, 2014.

26. Abelson, R. Whistle-blower suit says device maker generously rewards doctors. *New York Times*, January 24, 2006: C1.

27. Carreyrou, J, McGinty, T. Taking double cut, surgeons implant their own devices. *Wall Street Journal*, October 8, 2011: A1.

28. Kahn, CN. Intolerable risk, irreparable harm: The legacy of physician-owned specialty hospitals. Health Affairs *(Millwood)* 25 (1): 130-133, 2006.

29. Luxenberg, S. Invest in a surgicenter? *Medical Economics*, December 5, 2003: 60-65.

30. Bach, PB. Paying doctors to ignore patients. *New York Times*, July 24, 2008.

31. Lotto, DL. The corporate takeover of the soul of healthcare. *J Psychohistory* 26

(2): 603-609, 1998.

32. Elliott, S. G.E. to spend $100 million promoting itself as innovative. *New York Times,* January 16, 2003: C1.

33. Greider, W. *Who Will Tell the People? The Betrayal of American Democracy.* New York. Simon & Schuster, 1992.

34. Action Alert. FAIR Fairness & Accuracy in Reporting. New York City. NBC slams universal health care. November 12, 2002.

35. Kent, M. Breaking down the barriers. *The Nation,* June 8, 1998:29.

36. Konrad, W. Think twice before signing up for that medical credit card. *New York Times*, November 27, 2010: B5.

37. Project of the ABIM Foundation. ACP-ASIM Foundation and European Federation of Internal Medicine. Medical professionalism in the new millennium: A physician charter. *Ann Intern Med* 136 (3): 243-246, 2002.

38. Elliott, C. *White Coat Black Hat: Adventures on the Dark Side of Medicine.* Boston. Beacon Press, 2010: xi.

39. Pescasolido. BA, Tuch, SA, Martin, JA. The profession of medicine and the public: examining America's changing confidence in physician authority from the beginning of the "Health Care Crisis" to the era of health care reform. *J Health & Soc Behavior 42* (1): 1-16, 2001.

40. Schlesinger, M. A loss of faith: The sources of reduced political legitimacy for the American medical profession. *The Milbank Q* (80 (2): 185-235, 2002.

41. Friedman, E. Rocket science. *Health Forum Journal.* Spring 2003. Available at http://www.hospitalconnect.com/healthforumjournal/jsp/voices. jsp?voicepic=emily_pic

42. Ginsberg, C. The patient as profit center: Hospital Inc. comes to town. *The Nation,* November 18, 1996, p. 18.

43. Churchill, LR. Hegemony of money: Commercialism and professionalism in American medicine. *Cambridge Quarterly of Health Care*, Spring, 2007.

CHAPTER FIVE

OBAMACARE, THE CORPORATE "ALLIANCE" AND THE DIVERSION OF REFORM

The historical background from the last chapters makes it obvious that serious health care reform is needed. With the election of Barack Obama in the 2008 elections, his incoming administration had a great advantage—control of the White House and both houses of Congress. He declared on election night:

Change has come. This is our moment. This is our time . . . to reclaim the American Dream and reaffirm that fundamental truth—that out of many, we are one; that while we breathe, we hope, and where we are met with cynicism, and doubt, and those who tell us that we can't, we will respond with that timeless creed that sums up the spirit of a people: yes we can.[1]

So hope we did, and what then happened to health care reform? Unfortunately, his elegant words let us down as the central issues causing our system problems went unaddressed in the political compromises that soon followed.

This chapter has two objectives: (1) to briefly trace the rocky political road to passage of the Affordable Care Act in March, 2010; and (2) to recount how initial framing, lobbying, and corporate money foretold the outcome.

THE ROCKY ROAD TO PASSAGE

The 15 months of intense news coverage by the media, every day, led to a cliffhanger vote in Congress. It was a hard-fought battle full of political compromises that ended up with a bill serving private interests more than the public interest.

The Corporate "Alliance" of the Big Four

Disregarding, or unaware of history, Obama made the same mistake at the starting gate as the Clintons did in 1993—going to the corporate stakeholders, who are responsible for prices and costs of the health care system, for guidance in crafting reform.

Obama surrounded himself with corporate insiders who were part of the system problems, with conflicts of interest of their own. As one example, Nancy-Ann DeParle was brought in as White House director of the Office of Health Reform. She had received more than $6 million while serving on boards of directors of at least six companies that were targets of federal investigations, whistleblower lawsuits, or other regulatory actions.[2]

In May of 2009, four months after his inauguration, the new president held a high-profile event in the White House, convening representatives from the insurance, drug, medical device and hospital industries, together with business, labor and organized medicine, to a meeting to discuss health care reform. That was to end up as a fox-in-the-henhouse approach.

From that meeting, a so-called "alliance" was formed of the major stakeholders in the medical-industrial complex in favor of health care reform. A *voluntary* commitment was made to reduce health care costs by 1.5 percent, or some $1 trillion over the next ten years. Participants agreed to "cut both overuse and underuse of health care by aligning quality and efficiency initiatives." The White House quickly hailed this day as an "historic day, a watershed event, because these savings will help to achieve comprehensive health care reform."[3] Two months later, after this initial "charm offensive" of the major players, President Obama thought he had real momentum toward real reform, stating in a Rose Garden briefing that:

> ... *the fact that we have made so much progress where we've got doctors, nurses, hospitals, even the pharmaceutical industry, AARP, saying this makes sense to do, I think means*

that the stars are aligned and we need to take advantage of that.[4]

It soon became clear that the Big Four—the insurance, drug and hospital industries, together with organized medicine, were to script much of whatever bill would go forward. Let's take each in order to see what their agendas and tactics were as they entered the ring.

Insurers

The insurance industry initially appeared to be flexible and cooperative. Karen Ignagni, the CEO of the industry's trade group, America's Health Insurance Plans (AHIP), accepted the premise that "the system is not working today and needs to be reformed." If all Americans were to be required to buy health insurance, the industry would abandon pre-existing conditions as an underwriting principle, accept all applicants for insurance, and stop charging women higher premiums than men; at the same time, sick people would pay more for coverage than the healthy.[5]

The insurance industry was anticipating up to 50 million new enrollees in a greatly expanded market, and could afford to be cooperative in the early stages. But after the charm offensive, the industry lobbied hard in its own self-interest by:

- Vigorously opposing any public option as an effort to bring competition to the market, claiming that it could not be a level playing field and would put them out of business;
- Opposing any controls or caps on premium rates;
- Fighting against any cuts in overpayments to Medicare Advantage plans or attempts to set medical loss ratios too high (the lower they are, the more insurers gain);
- Lobbying in favor of setting the lowest possible minimal standards for insurance coverage; and
- Launching ad campaigns to tell the public how the industry is doing its part to support health care reform.[6]

The Drug Industry

As the CEO of PhRMA (Pharmaceutical Research and Manufacturers of America), Billy Tauzin was an old hand at politics for the drug industry. Six years earlier, the former Democrat turned Republican Congressman from Louisiana had played a leading role as chairman of a House committee in the design and passage of the Medicare Prescription Drug, Improvement and Modernization Act of 2003 (MMA). That legislation turned the prescription drug benefit over to the private sector and prohibited the government from negotiating drug prices. Tauzin then went through the revolving door between government, K Street and industry, including a stint as a top lobbyist in Washington, D.C., with a reported salary of about $2 million a year, lobbying against price controls and importation of drugs from other countries.[7] In an agreement with the president and Senator Max Baucus (D-Mont), chairman of the Senate Finance Committee, the drug industry came up early with a voluntary pledge of $80 billion toward health care reform in exchange for 12 more years of patent protection. Wall Street and investors loved that as stock prices rose by five to eight percent in the next month.[8]

Then competing bills in Congress led the industry to a flurry of actions to defend itself against government price controls, which were included in a House bill. It launched an ad campaign through a front group, deceptively named Americans for Stable Quality Care[9], and raised drug prices by 9 percent over the previous year; that increase more than covered the cost of the industry's first-year installment on its ten-year $80 billion pledge.[10]

Hospital industry

After the insurance and drug industries offered up their voluntary pledges toward the costs of health care reform, the hospital industry found itself needing to keep its place at the negotiating table. The stakes soon increased when the Obama administration proposed to cut payments to hospitals by $224 billion over the next ten years to help fund reform.[11] A "preliminary agreement" was soon struck with the White House and Senate Finance Committee pledging that the hospital industry would voluntarily accept cuts in Medicare and Medicaid payments by $155 billion over the next ten years.[12]

Together with the insurance and drug industries, the hospital industry's pledge would have been more than offset by expanded markets through the mandates of Obamacare. But the hospital industry did not speak with one voice. As one example, general hospitals were pitted against physician and investor-owned specialty hospitals. A major study had already determined that "specialty hospitals are contributing to a medical arms race without demonstrating clear quality advantages."[13]

Meanwhile, while supporting the general concept of health care reform, the hospital industry was playing both sides of the street—lobbying behind the scenes against cuts in Medicare reimbursement and other potential adverse impacts on its financial bottom line.

Organized medicine

Recall that the AMA has opposed any move toward universal health care since 1917. It was also against Medicare until the American Hospital Association and Blue Cross supported it in the 60s.[14] This time around, it made no specific pledge toward reform, but lent its qualified support for reform after the Administration offered a $245 billion "doc fix" in physician reimbursement over ten years.

Again, the AMA and most medical organizations came across as more interested in their future reimbursement than public policy. They vigorously opposed the public option as a threat to private insurers[15], opposed an empowered independent Medicare rate-setting commission[16] and an administration proposal to cut Medicare payments to cardiologists and oncologists while raising payments for family physicians and nurses.[17] When a 5 percent tax on elective cosmetic surgery became part of a Senate bill, it was dubbed the "Botax" after the anti-wrinkle product Botox. The AMA called the tax the first federal levy against a medical procedure[18] while the American Academy of Cosmetic Surgery opposed it as a tax against women and the baby boomer generation.[19] So much for the medical profession's leadership in health policy in the public interest.

Table 5.1 summarizes the pledges, agendas, tactics and anticipated rewards for each of the Big Four in the Corporate "Alliance."

How the "Alliance" was not an alliance

Although the Big Four were united in wanting to grow their markets through a larger population of insured people, while avoiding burdensome regulation along the way, that's about as far as the "alliance" went. Most of the time, their interests diverged to the point that they were hardly partners. They battled each other, each blaming another for being the culprit of higher costs—in effect, a circular firing squad. Examples include insurers fighting physicians' high out-of-network fees, while medical organizations were suing insurers for non-payment of fees. As president of the consulting firm Health Policy & Strategy Associates, Robert Laszewski observed:

It's always someone else's fault. There is not an incentive for these people to cooperate because the game they are playing is getting a bigger piece of the pie.[20]

As momentum for some kind of a reform bill gathered steam, Bob Herbert, well-known columnist for the *New York Times*, wrote:

The drug companies, the insurance industry and the rest of the corporate high-rollers have their tentacles all over this so-called reform effort, squeezing it for all its worth. Meanwhile, the public—struggling with the worst economic downturn since the 1930s—is looking on with great anxiety and confusion. If the drug companies and the insurance industry are smiling, it can only mean that the public interest is being left behind.[21]

TABLE 5.1

CORPORATE "ALLIANCE" FOR HEALTH CARE REFORM - THE BIG FOUR

Insurance Industry

Pledge	Abandon pre-existing conditions as an underwriting principle
	Accept all applicants
	Stop charging women higher premiums than men
Agenda	Grow private and public insurance markets by up to 50 million enrollees
Tactics	Oppose controls or caps on premium rates
	Oppose the public option
	Lobby for low standards for insurance coverage and low MLRs
	Fight against cuts of overpayments for Medicare Advantage plans
Rewards	Larger private and public markets
	Higher profits and returns to shareholders
	Preempt increased regulation by government

PhRMA

Pledge	$80 billion over 10 years toward costs of health care reform
Agenda	Expand private and public markets
	Avoid price controls and competition from importation of drugs from other countries
	Gain maximal patent protection for biotech drugs
Tactics	With assurance from White House agreement that government would not negotiate drug prices or import drugs from abroad, lobbied jointly with Families USA in support of health care reform as represented by bills in Congress
Rewards	Expanded private and public markets
	Higher profits and returns to shareholders
	Avoid increased regulation by government

Hospital Industry

Pledge	$155 billion over 10 years in reduced hospital charges
Agenda	Growth in future revenues in private and public markets
Tactics	Lobby for employer and individual mandates, and expansion of Medicaid
Rewards	Larger private and public markets
	Increased revenues ($170 billion), more than offsetting its pledged amount (40)

Organized Medicine

Pledge	No specific pledge
Agenda	Support private markets and restrain government intervention
	Prevent cuts in Medicare reimbursement
Tactics	Supports employer and individual mandates, insurance reforms, and expansion of Medicaid
	Opposes public option, rate-setting by independent commission, and targeted reimbursement cuts by specialty
Rewards	$245 billion "doc fix" restores Medicare reimbursement, at least for a time
	Increased revenues from expanded insured population

Source: Geyman, JP *Hijacked: The Road to Single-Payer In the Aftermath of Stolen Health Care Reform*. Friday Harbor, WA. Copernicus Healthcare, 2010, p.30

As we shall soon see, the pump was primed to the Big Four and other corporate interests in the medical-industrial complex to get as much as possible out of a reform bill—for their own gains, but at the expense of patients and taxpayers.

The Battle of Bills and Distortion to the End Game

The House took the early lead in developing reform bills by merging three of its committees into one. Without going into details, it called for an individual mandate, an employer mandate, health insurance exchanges, a public option, an essential benefits package, subsidies for individuals and employers, various insurance reforms, expansion of Medicaid, and a new Center for Comparative Effectiveness Research. Then the Senate came up with two bills, the second of which drew the most attention and attacks from both the right and left—the bill crafted behind closed doors of the Senate Finance Committee, chaired by Senator Max Baucus (D-MT). Immediately labeled the "Baucus bill," it had some similarities with the other bills. But it had some major differences from the House bill and the other Senate bill, especially in dropping the public option and excluding abortion as a covered benefit.[22]

Although the House had a large Democratic majority (256-178) and the Senate had a potentially filibuster-proof majority of 60 (58 Democrats and 2 Independents), the battle went down to the wire from the summer of 2009 to final passage on March 25, 2010. Distortion and demagoguery took over through town hall meetings during the August congressional recess. Conservatives and their well-funded organizations on the right sought to defeat any reform bill, charging that it would be a government takeover, lead to socialized medicine, restrict choice, bring higher taxes, and invoke "death panels." Just leave health care to the free market, was the message loud and clear. Recall Rick Scott from the last chapter, who was fired from Columbia/HCA after the huge federal fraud settlement. Here he is again as founder and head of Conservatives for Patients' Rights, declaring that:

72

Any serious discussion of health care reform that does not include choice, competition, accountability and responsibility—the four 'pillars' of patients' rights—will result in our government truly becoming a 'nanny state,' making decisions based on what is best for society and government rather than individuals deciding what is best for each of us."[23]

Fast forward to the end game after months of intense debate and hundreds of amendments to various bills in both chambers of Congress. It soon became clear that the Big Four would get what they wanted. As examples, the insurance industry saw the public option killed while the drug industry cheered a Senate vote 51-48 against a provision that would have allowed importation of cheaper prescription drugs from Canada and some other countries.[24]

Faced with final votes in Congress that could go either way after all these months, President Obama caved once more in his "This is it" speech on March 3, 2010, even as he denigrated Medicare and gave fuel to his opponents on the right:[25]

On one end of the spectrum, there are some who have suggested scrapping our system of private insurance and replacing it with government-run health care. Though many countries have such a system, in America it would be neither practical nor realistic . . . I don't believe we should give government bureaucrats or insurance company bureaucrats more control over health care in America.

Matthew Rothschild, editor of *The Progressive* quickly responded:

By damning 'government bureaucrats,' Obama played right into the hands of the anti-government crowd and made any durable expansion of health care coverage all the more difficult. He also cast aspersions on every single federal employee in the Medicare and Medicaid and VA and Indian health programs. Single-payer advocates like you and me were props for him all along.

Finally, the Affordable Care Act became law on March 25, 2010, with these votes:

- In the House, on March 21: by 219-212
- In the Senate, on March 24: by 56-43
- In the House again, on March 25: by 220-207.

The long journey was over, but the fireworks over it were not!

HOW HEALTH CARE REFORM WAS DIVERTED

Among the various factors that led to the ramping down of the potential effectiveness of this iteration of health care reform, these stand out.

Flawed framing of the issues

Despite newly attained control of both chambers in Congress and the White House, the Democrats took a timid approach to framing the issues, essentially ruling out single-payer as not politically feasible. They accepted without critique some bogus "research" conclusions of Celinda Lake, a self-described "leading political strategist" for the Democratic Party, who concluded that Americans think Medicare is "frighteningly flawed", that they don't want universal coverage, and that activists should say "choice of public and private plans" instead of "Medicare-for-all." Her polling had been based on giving respondents two choices— "guaranteed affordable choice" or single-payer. Her "findings" contradicted the results of many legitimate national studies over the years that 65 to 85 percent of Americans support universal health insurance, and that 60 to 70 percent support single-payer Medicare-for-all.[26] In effect, this was a "Surrender in Advance" strategy that bailed out the private insurance industry from the get-go.

On the right, Republicans accepted the recommendations of Frank Luntz, a political consultant and pollster, that they stress such words as "rationing", "takeover", and "bureaucrats." Their messaging was without substance, calling for "patient-centered reforms", "common-sense simple fixes, not politically-driven experiments", and "a bottom-up, patient-centered system where control remains with your doctor and you."[27]

Both frames were completely off target in not focusing on major system problems and being uninformed by health policy science or the track record of previous incremental reform attempts. Republican framing was mostly untrue and based on scare words. Democrats tried to sell their vision of reform as letting people "keep your insurance if you like it."[28]

Corruption of the political process

Corporate stakeholders in our market-based system had many ways to guide, even control, whatever health reform bill would come out of Congress. As the debate heated up in 2009, lobbyists descended on Washington, D.C., like locusts. By August of that year, there were 3,300 registered lobbyists representing more than 1,500 organizations working on the health care issue. Thousands of other unregistered lobbyists were also involved.[29] As Bill Allison, a senior fellow at the Sunshine Foundation observed:

> *When you have a big piece of legislation like this, it's like ringing the dinner bell for K Street . . . There's a lot of money at stake and there are a lot of special interests who don't want their ox gored.*[30]

Larry McNeely, a health care advocate with the Boston-based U.S. Public Interest Research Group, said:

> *The sheer quantity of money that's sloshed around Washington is drowning out the voices of citizens and the groups that speak up for them.*[31]

A February 2010 analysis by the Center for Public Integrity found that more than 1,750 companies and organizations had hired about 4,525 lobbyists—eight for every member of Congress—to influence health care legislation in 2009.[32] Successful lobbyists could later find their own verbatim words issued as press statements from legislators whom they had targeted. By the time that the bill was finally passed, the lobbying industry had taken in $1.2 *billion*.[33] Figure 5.1 illustrates what was going on.

FIGURE 5.1

No Solutions in Sight

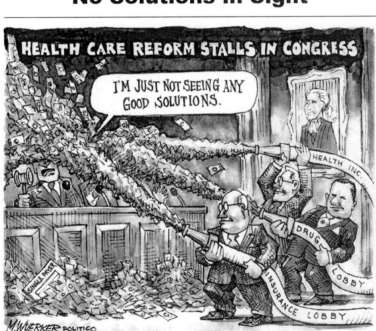

Reprinted with permission from Matt Wuerker of Politico.

Three examples illustrate how specific these lobbying efforts were:

- Tim Trysla, executive director of the Access to Medical Imaging Coalition (note the wording!) lobbied 120 legislators, sometimes together with General Electric representatives, arguing against any cuts in reimbursement for CT and MRI scans.[34]

- The Community Oncology Alliance (again note the wording) spent $200,000 on lobbyists in the second quarter of 2009, and brought 100 oncologists to Capitol Hill to demand that proposed cuts in Medicare reimbursement to oncologists be reversed. (Oncologists had been receiving lucrative kickbacks from drug companies for administering cancer drugs).[35]
- The 33 lobbyists deployed by the AMA successfully killed the proposed tax on cosmetic surgery.[36]

Health care industries targeted both political parties in their lobbying, especially those best placed to shape the health reform bills. Senator Max Baucus, as chairman of the powerful Senate Finance Committee (SFC), was a primary target. Campaign contributions, of course, were an important part of the influence peddling process. He led the pack among the 23 members of the SFC with $1,148,775 in 2008 alone and $2,797,381 over his career from the health sector plus a career total of another $1,170,313 from the insurance industry, according to the Center for Responsive Politics.[37]

As a key shaper of the final health reform legislation, Baucus had his own additional conflicts of interest, mostly below the radar and not reported by the mainstream media. He appointed Elizabeth Fowler as his "chief operating officer" for health reform. She was an insurance industry insider, having served as vice president of public policy for WellPoint, the country's largest health insurer, from 2006 to 2008. She was widely recognized as the lead author of the SFC health reform bill.[38]

Predictably the public option was killed in the SFC, and the single-payer alternative was never considered. It is an ugly story—the Baucus Eight incident. In May 2009, when a hearing of health reform options was to be held before his committee, single-payer activists organized call-in days and faxes to committee members well in advance of the meeting, requesting one seat at the table of 15 for an advocate of a single-payer national health plan. After many hundreds of calls and faxes, no response was received until the day before the event, when they were told that no more invitations would be issued for what was also billed as a "public roundtable discussion." On the day of the meeting, eight activists entered the chambers and made their request known. Baucus's immediate response—"We need more police." All eight were arrested, handcuffed, charged with disorderly conduct and disrupting a congressional hearing, and carted off to jail. Charges were later dropped, but some community service was required of the "offenders." Some media reported the story, including MSNBC, which featured Dr. Margaret Flowers, a pediatrician and member of Physicians for a National Health Program, as the leading story shortly thereafter on *The Ed Show*.[39]

Big money and the media

The mainstream media are now mostly owned by large corporate interests that to an increasing extent are bought and paid for by industry. The corporate reach of today's "journalism" extends to all forms of media, including print, digital, radio, and television. We can put "journalism" in quotes these days as investigative reporting declines for lack of funding and as corporate media offer "information" masquerading as news. In their excellent 2010 book, Robert McChesney and John Nichols warn that:

> *This is not a routine crisis. It fundamentally brings to a head the long-simmering tension between journalism and commerce.*[40]

There are many ways whereby the corporate media are for sale and receptive to spinning the news in the interest of sponsoring stakeholders without disclosure of conflicts of interest. Here are just some of them, of which most of us are unaware.

Corporate media catering to industry

Katherine Weymouth, an attorney, graduate of the Harvard School of Business, and publisher of the *Washington Post,* decided to raise some cash during the mid-summer health care debate

78

in 2009. A scheme was launched to host a dozen off-the-record "salons" at her Washington, D.C. home. Lobbyists, politicians, and invited members from the Obama administration were to be convened to discuss health care policy with some of her editors and reporters. Each of these private dinner parties would have a maximal attendance of twenty. Invitees were offered sponsorship of an individual salon for $25,000 or an annual series sponsorship of 11 salons for $250,000. A promotional flyer stated that: [This is] "an exclusive opportunity to participate in the health care reform debate among the select few who will actually get it done. . . A unique opportunity for stakeholders to hear and be heard."

When this plan became known, a firestorm of protest led to its cancellation and a public relations disaster for the paper.[41] But that was just one example of similar arrangements taken by other major news outlets.

Interlocking directorates

Interlocking directorates are more the rule than the exception throughout the corporate media industry. When directors of one corporation sit on other corporate boards, conflicts of interest are common, especially when editors and journalists are called upon to report stories that will likely result in loss of revenue to their employers. A 2009 study by Fairness & Accuracy in Reporting (FAIR) looked at the connections between nine major media corporations and their major outlets—Disney (ABC), General Electric (NBC), Time Warner (CNN, *Time)*, News Corporation (Fox), New York Times Co., Washington Post Co. (*Newsweek*), Tribune Co. (*Chicago Tribune, Los Angeles Times*) and Gannett (*USA Today)*—there were board connections to six different insurance companies in this group, while six of the nine media corporations had such connections with pharmaceutical companies. With such close ties to two of our Big Four, it comes as no surprise that single-payer national health insurance was barely mentioned as an alternative to the present system.[42]

Ties to conservative talk shows, writers, editors and book publishers

As we know, Rupert Murdoch is one of the biggest media power brokers in the world. His holdings include the Fox News Channel, *The Weekly Standard*, Dow Jones, and owner of the *Wall Street Journal*, as well as other news outlets.[43] These conservative publications consistently promote free markets with minimal regulation and no price controls. In health care, the message is freedom to choose our health care with little concern whether we can afford it or not. Eric Alterman, professor of journalism at the CUNY Graduate School of Journalism, describes Fox News as an extremist propaganda outlet, asking us to consider whether a bona fide news organization would, as Fox has done:

- "run, over a five-day period, twenty-two excerpts from healthcare forums in which every single speaker was opposed?
- allow a producer to cheer-lead, off camera, anti-Obama protesters?
- run these kinds of headlines, as a 'Fox Nation Victory': SENATE REMOVES 'END OF LIFE' PROVISION and CONGRESS DELAYS HEALTH CARE RATIONING BILL?"[44]

CONCLUDING COMMENTS

So there you have it. That is how Obamacare, the ACA, came into being. A shoddy political process, with the debate and votes in Congress hijacked by the Big Four and their allies. Lawrence Lessig, professor of law at Harvard Law School and author of the excellent 2011 book *Republic, Lost: How Money Corrupts Congress—and a Plan to Stop It*, sums up the problem this way:

We don't have real financial reform, because millions have been spent to protect bloated banks. We don't have

*real health care reform, because the insurance companies
and pharmaceutical companies had the power to veto
any real change to the insanely inefficient status quo. . .
. Our Congress is politically corrupt. It struts around as
if all were fine, as if it deserved the honor that its
auspicious Capitol building inspires. It acts as if nothing
were wrong. As if the people didn't notice.*[45]

It is time to move on to Part Two to see what the ACA really
brings us beyond the hype and promises.

References

1.   Obama, B. Transcript: Obama's acceptance speech. Election night. Chicago, Il. *Yahoo News*, November 4, 2008.
2.   MSNBC. Obama health czar directed firms in trouble: http://www.msnbc.msn.com/id/31566399/ns/health-health_care/
3.   Pear, R. Health care's early pledges. *New York Times*, May 12, 2009: A1.
4.   Koffler, K. The Rose Garden: Administration exaggerates alliances on reform. *Roll Call*, July 27, 2009.
5.   Meckler, L, Fuhrmans, V. Insurers offer to end prices tied to illness. *Wall Street Journal*, March 25, 2009: A4.
6.   Geyman, JP. *Hijacked: The Road to Single-payer in the Aftermath of Stolen Health Care Reform*. Monroe, ME. Common Courage Press, 2010:10.
7.   Lueck, S. Tauzin is named top lobbyist for pharmaceutical industry. *Wall Street Journal*, December 16, 2004: A4.
8.   Adamy, J, Hitt, G. CEOs tally health-bill score. *Wall Street Journal*, October 19, 2009: A3.
9.   Murray, M. PhRMA-funded ads tout health care reform. *Roll Call*, November 23, 2009.
10. Wilson, D. Drug companies increase prices in face of change. *New York Times*, November 16, 2009: A1.
11. Adamy, J, Rockoff, JD. Hospital industry bristles at cuts. *Wall Street Journal*, June 15, 2009: A3.
12. Medicare Rights Center. White House announces deal with hospitals to cut Medicare and Medicaid payments. *Medicare Watch*, issue 14, July 15, 2009.
13. Berenson, RA, Bazzoli, FGJ, Au, M. Do specialty hospitals promote price competition? Center for Studying Health System Change. Issue Brief No. 103, January, 2006.

14. Marmor, TR. *The Politics of Medicare.* New York. Aldine Publishing Company, 1970, pp 27-31.
15. Pear, R. Doctors' group opposes public health insurance plan. *New York Times,* June 11, 2009: A17.
16. Goldstein, J. Doctors oppose giving commission power over Medicare payments. *Wall Street Journal,* July 29, 2009: A3.
17. Nussbaum. A, Rapaport, L. Cardiologists crying foul over Obama Medicare cuts (Update 1). *Bloomberg News,* August 28, 2009.
18. Rockoff, JD. Knives drawn over 'Botox'. *Wall Street Journal,* December 4, 2009: A3.
19. Galewitz, P. Plastic surgeons cry foul over 'Botox' proposal in Senate health bill. *Kaiser Health News.* November 20, 2009.
20. Johnson, A. Race to pin blame for health costs. *Wall Street Journal,* February 10, 2010: A5.
21. Herbert, B. This is reform? *New York Times,* August 17, 2009.
22. Hitt, G, Adamy, J, Weisman, J. Senate bill sets lines for health showdown. *Wall Street Journal,* September 17, 2009: A1.
23. Web site for Conservatives for Patients' Rights, accessed October 5, 2009.
24. Mundy, A Drug-import bill rejected by Senate. *Wall Street Journal,* December 16, 2009: A7.
25. Rothschild, M. The Mary Ivins story. *The Progressive* 74 (4): April 2010.
26. Sullivan, K. An analysis of Celinda Lake's slide show: How to talk to voters about health care. November 29, 2008. Available at http://www.pnhp.org. news.2008/december/americans support si.php
27. Castellanos, A. GOP health care talking points. July 7, 2009. As cited by the *Washington Post,* July 20, 2009.
28. Ibid # 6: 61-71.
29. Kroll, A. Lobbyists still run Washington. *The Progressive Populist,* October 15, 2009.
30. Salant, JD, O'Leary, L. Six lobbyists per lawmaker work on health overhaul. *Bloomberg News,* as cited in *Truthout,* August 17, 2009.
31. Ibid # 30.
32. Eaton, J, Pell, MB. Lobbyists swarm capitol to influence health reform. Washington, D.C. The Center for Public Integrity, February 23, 2010.
33. Center for Public Integrity, as cited in Moyers, B, Winship, M. The unbearable lightness of reform. *Truthout,* March 27, 2010.
34. Adamy, J, Williamson, E. As Congress goes on break, health lobbying heats up. *Wall Street Journal,* August 5, 2009: A1.
35. Meropol, NJ, Schulman, KA. Cost of cancer care: Issues and implications. *J Clin Oncology* 25: 180-186, 2007.
36. Ibid # 34.
37. Editorial. Puppets in Congress. *New York Times,* November 17, 2009: A28.
38. Conner, K. Chief health aide to Baucus is former Wellpoint executive. *Eyes on the Ties* blog, September 1, 2009.
39. Robbins, K. Baucus 8 update: Single-payer in the news. Healthcare-NOW! May 7, 2009. Available at http://www.healthcare-now.org/Baucus-8-update-single-payer-in...

40. McChesney, R, Nichols, J. *The Death and Life of American Journalism.* Philadelphia. Nation Books, 2010, p 2.
41. Allen, M, Calderone, M. *Washington Post* cancels lobbyist event amid uproar. *Truthout,* July 2, 2009.
42. Murphy, K. Single-payer & interlocking directorates. *Extra!,* August 2009, p 7.
43. Wikipedia, listing for Rupert Murdoch, accessed October 17, 2009.
44. Alterman, E. Just don't call it "journalism". *The Nation* 289 (15): 10, November 9, 2009.
45. Lessig, L. *Republic, Lost: How Money Corrupts Congress—and a Plan to Stop It.* New York. Twelve. 2011: 246-247.

Part Two

A FIVE-YEAR EXPERIENCE WITH OBAMACARE

CHAPTER 6

THE AFFORDABLE CARE ACT:
PROMISES VS. REALITIES

With Obamacare the law of the land for almost five years, about halfway through its legislative life, we can now start to take stock of what it has done and is likely to accomplish. It is time to ask whether it will effectively address the Big Four challenges of health care reform—restricted access, uncontrolled increases in costs, increasing unaffordability, and variable, often mediocre quality of care.

Having traced in the last chapter the intense national debate and tortuous path the ACA had through Congress, it is worth recalling ten major promises made by the Obama administration and its supporters along the way. This chapter has one simple goal: to recall ten of these promises and assess to what extent they have, or are likely to be met.

TEN PROMISES OF THE OBAMA ADMINISTRATION

1. Health care reform will be negotiated in public view.

In a town hall meeting on August 21, 2008, Obama promised televised negotiations for the health care law.[1] But, as we have already seen, most of the negotiations were in private and closely held until participants announced their agreements to the public. Alternatives for discussion were restricted to the interests of the major corporate stakeholders.

The single-payer alternative, for example, was never on the table. The reasons are simple enough, but they are under the radar. As Lawrence Lessig, whom we met in the last chapter, points out:

Influence can be exercised—and hence a campaign contribution rewarded—in any of the stages of the potential life of a bill. If it is, it is invisible to the regressions. . . . In a whole host of ways, legislative power can be exercised without a trace, the regressions cannot map cause and effect. As the House Select Committee on Lobbying Activities describes, 'Complex government inevitably means government with bottlenecks at which pressure can be quietly and effectively applied. . . The prevention of government action, and this is the aim of many lobbies, is relatively easy under these circumstances.' [2]

Concerning the single-payer alternative, even some Republicans might have voted for it. Larry Pressler, former Republican senator from South Dakota from 1979 to 1997, commented on this subject in 2011:

There should have been an up or down vote on [single-payer health insurance], or a vote at least on cloture. There was neither. For some reason, it just went away. Barack Obama abandoned it completely, although he had said he was for it. Some Republicans are for it—I was for it way back and Nixon was for it . . . on a much more significant basis. Bob Packwood had a plan for it. But the point is, when they really started doing the health care bill, I would suspect that is because of the insurance companies' contributions, especially to the Democrats. [3]

Exactly right. The three largest insurers, together with America's Health Insurance Plans (AHIP), the industry's trade group, contributed more than $7 million dollars in campaign funding in 2007-2008, targeted at those legislators best positioned to shape the health care law. Those up for re-election in 2010 received $23 million for their campaign war chests by October 2009. [4]

2. If you like your insurance, you can keep it.

In a talk at the annual meeting of the American Medical Association on June 15, 2009, President Obama said this about the Affordable Care Act:

> *So let me begin by saying this to you and to the American people: I know that there are millions of Americans who are content with their health care coverage—they like their plan and, most importantly, they value their relationship with their doctor. They trust you. And that means that no matter how we reform health care, we will keep this promise to the American people: If you like your doctor, you will be able to keep your doctor, period. . . . If you like your health care plan, you'll be able to keep your health care plan, period. . . . No one will take it away, no matter what.*[5]

This promise was not credible from the outset. At best, it was naive and uninformed. Fact-checker PolitiFact.com, 2009 Pulitzer Prize awardee for National Reporting, called this its 2013 Lie of the Year.

There are many reasons that made this promise impossible to keep. For openers, the ACA grandfathered in all employer-sponsored policies from the get-go, so that they are exempted from any insurance reforms under the ACA until 2018. And as we have known for years, there are many ways whereby people insured by their employers can lose their coverage—ranging from changing or losing their job to employers cutting employees back to part-time to employers withdrawing coverage or making it unaffordable. Recent experience with employer-sponsored insurance (ESI) has shown that employers increasingly offer higher deductible plans to keep their costs down, thereby shifting more costs to their employees. David Cusano, a senior research fellow at Georgetown University, has this comment about the increasing financial insecurity of people with ESI coverage:

> *The question now becomes, 'Can I afford to use it?' When you think about people confronting out-of-pocket*

maximums at around $7,000 or deductibles of $5,000 for a family, that's a lot of money. You throw in prescription drug copays into the mix, and I can see where you would be worried.[6]

There are other ways by which ESI is unstable and undependable since the ACA became law. In an effort to avoid federal penalties of about $2,000 per employee for not offering health insurance, some large employers with at least 50 employees, are offering barebones, "skinny" plans that cover preventive care but not such major benefits as hospital care. Premiums for such policies cost about one-half as much as for plans with hospital coverage—good for the employer but not for employees, who are barred from getting federal subsidies through the ACA's exchanges.[7] It is an embarrassment to the Obama administration that an online spreadsheet developed by the Department of Health and Human Services developed a calculator for employers to use that allowed plans to exclude hospital coverage. In an effort to close this loophole, the Obama administration announced in November 2014 that it will issue regulations in 2015 to ban large employers from qualifying health plans under the ACA that don't include coverage for hospital care.[8] Another way that employers can get around federal penalties is by enrolling their employees in Medicaid plans; this option has been taken by a number of employers with lower-wage workers, such as in the food industry.[9]

Where the ACA does kick in—in the small business and individual markets—the promise of keeping your insurance if you like, often does not hold. The ACA grandfathered in health plans in the individual market that were in place when the bill was enacted in 2010, whether or not they met the new ACA standards. In 2013, as the January 2014 implementation date loomed for these standards to kick in, many thousands of people received notices that their coverage was being cancelled. Some insurers were notifying their policyholders that they would have to change plans, while others were discontinuing 20 percent of their individual business. Some of the cancellations were for plans that did not meet the ACA's standards for coverage, such as a Florida Blue policy that did not cover ER visits or hospitalizations and paid only $50 toward physician visits. Other policies were cancelled when the insurer discontinued whole categories of coverage.[10] People losing coverage were often offered new policies that would meet the ACA's requirements, but the premium hikes for many were unaffordable.[11]

Fast forward to October 2014, and we find that cancelled policies are still a problem. Tens of thousands of people in many parts of the country are receiving notices from their insurers that their health plans are being cancelled. These insurers include Anthem (the largest), Humana in Louisville, KY, Health Care Services Corporation in Chicago, CareFirst in Baltimore, MD, and Kaiser Permanente in Oakland, CA. One reason for these cancellations is that insurers are finding that they can make more money selling plans that meet ACA requirements and qualify for federal subsidies for their higher premiums.[12]

3. If you like your doctor, you can keep your doctor.

There are many trends that have been working for some years against continuity of care with the same physician. But the ACA has accelerated these trends to the point that many patients cannot stay with their primary care physician or specialist, no matter how much they would like to. We are now seeing a new round of disruption throughout the health care system as planning for accountable care organizations (ACOs) goes forward, as hospital systems grow and consolidate, typically taking ownership of large physician groups, and as insurers compete by narrowing their networks of hospitals and physicians. More than one-half of U.S. physicians are now employed by other organizations, mostly hospital systems but also now by some insurers moving into the delivery side of health care. Networks can change at a moment's notice, based on business decisions of hospital systems or insurers, without any input from physicians or patients.

Here are two examples that illustrate how fragmented our "system" has become:

- The University of Pittsburgh Medical Center (UPMC) sent certified letters in late 2013 to several hundred patients informing them that they could no longer see their physicians. Some patients were cut off from their UPMC physicians even in the middle of cancer treatment. This was because their insurance, Community Blue, sold by Highmark, had become both a rival hospital system and an insurer.[13]
- As the biggest player in the Medicare Advantage market, UnitedHealthGroup Inc. has almost 3 million members and 350,000 physicians in its networks. Over the last months of 2013, it dropped thousands of physicians from its networks in at least ten states. Some 2,500 cancer patients at Moffitt Cancer Center in Tampa, Florida, were forced to switch plans or find other physicians.[14]

4. We will have a public option to put competitive pressure on insurers.

> *If you don't like your health care coverage or you don't have any insurance at all you'll have a chance, under what we've proposed, to take part in what we're calling a Health Insurance Exchange. This exchange will allow you to one-stop shop for a health care plan, compare benefits and prices, and choose a plan that's best for you and your family. . . . one of these options needs to be a public option that will give people a broader range of choices . . . and inject competition into the health care market so that we can force waste out of the system and keep the insurance companies honest.[15]*

This promise drew wide support from liberals but was strongly opposed by conservatives as likely to put private insurers out of business. The Congressional Budget Office (CBO) estimated that a public option would "save the government around $150 billion."[16] But Obama did not fight hard for the public option, later blaming Congress for failing to include it in the ACA, and giving in to the pressure and money of the insurance industry as he had to that of the drug industry. Although Obama's campaign rhetoric had included a goal to take on the special interests and to change the way Washington works, that is certainly not what happened. As Glenn Greenwald observed:

> *The way this bill has been shaped is the ultimate expression—and bolstering—of how Washington has long worked. One can find reasonable excuses for why it had to be done that way, but one cannot reasonably deny that it was.*[17]

5. If you are already insured, your insurance will be stronger, better and more secure than before.

From the start, nothing in the law guarantees that people can keep the health insurance that they had when the ACA took effect. Costs can rise, benefits changed, and in some instances, policies cancelled. Employers can shift employees to the exchanges, as many have. Larger, self-insured employers were grandfathered in under the ACA without having to meet its requirements. As a result, they can and have shifted more costs of coverage to their employees, increasingly making coverage unaffordable. Despite the rhetoric accompanying the ACA's enactment by its proponents, security of health insurance coverage was never in the cards.[18]

As we will see in forthcoming chapters, we are seeing an epidemic of *underinsurance,* accelerated under the ACA, among those who have insurance, whether through employers, the exchanges, or Medicaid. Here are some markers of the severity of this problem:

- Almost one-third of low-income (0-125 percent of federal poverty level) families spend more than 5 percent of their meager incomes on medical expenses, while many forego or delay necessary care or medications because of costs.[19]
- Nearly 1.2 million families seek bankruptcy protection each year, with medical bills the cause in two-thirds of cases, despite 75 percent of those bankrupted having been insured at the start of their illness or accident.[20]

- People gaining coverage through the exchanges most often select silver plans with actuarial values of only 70 percent, leaving enrollees responsible for 30 percent of health care costs.
- Many states have reduced Medicaid coverage, cut provider payments, and narrowed provider networks, thereby limiting access.[21]
- Figure 6.1 graphically shows the adverse impacts of underinsurance on the underinsured as compared to the insured and uninsured.

FIGURE 6.1

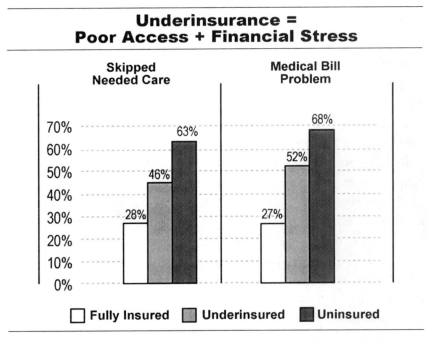

**Underinsurance =
Poor Access + Financial Stress**

Source: Reprinted with permission from The Commonwealth Fund. Skipped Rx, test, treatment, followup, or visit because of cost. September, 2011.

6. The website is simple and user-friendly.

This is what Health and Human Services (HHS) Secretary Kathleen Sebelius predicted about the ACA's website Healthcare. gov.[22] The Obamacare website opened on October 1, 2013, for the business of enrolling applicants for the health care exchanges which started in January 2014. Within days, its problems had become a media frenzy, a public relations disaster for the Obama administration, and a probable campaign issue during the 2014 election cycle. Just a few days into the website's rollout, it was out of order with widespread complaints. A new administrator was brought in, and there was plenty of blame to go around. The government was blamed for inadequate design and lack of oversight. Insurers complained that they were not getting the information they needed. Signups were falling far short of projections.

These problems were far from being fixed by the end of the signup period. A *Washington Post* report in early February found that 22,000 people had filed appeals to HHS to fix errors in their health insurance coverage caused by the website's glitches. As the website serving Obamacare exchanges in 36 states, it was failing to correctly calculate subsidies they were eligible for, often putting them into the wrong insurance program, or completely denying them coverage. These appeals were transferred over to the Center for Medicare and Medicaid Services (CMS) for follow-up, but the computer program to process these appeals did not yet exist at the time![23]

As new efforts were being made in preparation for the second open enrollment period, involving expansion of the exchange to additional states and adding new features to verify the incomes of people eligible for federal subsidies, the Government Accountability Office (GAO) cautioned that there will still be "bumps" with the second rollout of the federal exchange.[24] With the second open enrollment period (starting November 15, 2014 and extending to February 15, 2015), the process remains complex, with experts predicting wide swings in prices and equal or more confusion this time around—and with just three months available to choose a new policy.[25]

Especially important to consumers shopping on the exchanges in year two, the website still lacks the tools to allow them to see which doctors and hospitals will be included in individual insurance plans.[26] Another problem with the website is that the system has no way to alert an insurer when their customers come back to the site and switch to a new insurer for 2015. Moreover, consumers who purchased plans in 2014 can find themselves automatically enrolled in those plans for 2015 when they no longer want them.[27] Despite the government's efforts to protect its website from security breaches, the GAO acknowledged that "weaknesses remain in the security and privacy protections applied to Healthcare.gov and its supporting systems."[28]

Dr. Philip Caper, internist and health policy expert, sums up the website's problems in this way:

> *[the website's problems] are far more serious than poor software design. They are baked into the law by its extreme complexity. . . . the ACA creates complex new law that perpetuates and reinforces the chaos and confusion of our hodgepodge of public and private insurance programs. Coverage and financial assistance continue to depend on an individual's employment status, income, place of residence, age, conjectures about future health status and many other factors, some of them subject to change with little or no warning and many impossible to predict.*[29]

7. The ACA is helping 17 million children who would be denied insurance because of pre-existing conditions.

Here again is an expansive and inaccurate number declared by the Obama administration. PolitiFact finds that the number was cherry-picked by HHS as the highest of an estimated range of 4 to 17 million, also noting that many of these hypothetical children already have insurance despite pre-existing conditions. PolitiFact estimates the true number of children who are uninsured due to pre-existing conditions is somewhere in the range between 160,000 and 1.1 million.[30]

8. The average family will save $2,500 under the ACA.

> *I will sign a universal health care bill into law by the end of my first term as president that will cover every American*

and cut the cost of a typical family's premium by up to $2,500 a year.[31]

Obama made this claim repeatedly during and after his first presidential campaign, but it was never based on evidence or an accurate calculation. David Cutler, professor of economics at Harvard University, who advised Obama during that campaign, later confirmed that this figure was intended to apply to *total health costs* for a family, not just premiums.[32] Those costs, of course, would include deductibles, co-payments and out-of-pocket costs. So the number was specious from the start. Moreover, given the uncertainties and complexities of the ACA, it was obviously impossible to know, in advance, if *any* savings would *ever* be seen by American families. Moreover, of course, the ACA would never bring us universal access to health care.

9. The ACA will keep health care costs down.

The president's Council of Economic Advisers has said this. It is true that national health care expenditures have slowed somewhat in recent years, but most experts agree that this has not been due to the ACA. Other factors are clearly at work, starting well before the advent of the ACA, including the economic recession, fiscal policy changes, and a slowdown in growth in Medicaid and Medicare.[33]

10. The ACA will cost about $900 billion over 10 years.

This estimate will certainly be far below the real costs, which are still unknown. The CBO already discredited it with a doubled estimate in May 2013 of $1.8 trillion.[34]

CONCLUDING COMMENT

The pattern of these promises is clear—they were not credible when made and greatly exaggerated projections for the ACA. Granted, the ACA is byzantine in its complexity and there are so many variables and uncertainties that no accurate future promises could have been made. But these promises amount to propaganda that helped to garner enough political support to pass a deeply flawed bill that evolved through a debate that was not informed by fundamentals of health policy and our experience over the last 30 years.

The next three chapters will show just how far off base these promises were in terms of access, costs and affordability, and quality of U.S. health care.

References

1. Holan, AD, Kliegman, J. 10 things Obamacare supporters say that aren't entirely true. *Truth-O-Meter*, October 2, 2013.
2. Lessig, L. *Republic, Lost: How Money Corrupts Congress, and a Plan to Stop It.* New York. Twelve, 2011: p 150.
3. Lawrence Lessig interview with Larry Pressler, June 16, 2011.
4. Kroll, A. Lobbyists still run Washington. *The Progressive Populist*, October 15, 2009.
5. Drobnic Holan, A. "Lie of the Year: If you like your health care plan, you can keep it." htpp://www.politifact.com/truth-o-meter/article/2013/dec/12/lie-of-the-year-if-you-like-your-health-care-plan-keep-it/). PolitiFact.com.
6. Macdonald, J. Worried about insurance? That's common. *Bankrate.com*, September 4, 2014.
7. Hancock, J. Administration signals doubts about calculator permitting plans without hospital benefits. *Kaiser Health News*, October 18, 2014.
8. Hancock, J. Obama administration closing health law loophole for plans without hospitalization. Kaiser Health News, November 4, 2014.
9. Mathews, AW, Jargon, J. Firms try to escape health penalties. *Wall Street Journal*, October 22, 2014: A1.
10. Appleby, J. Why insurers cancel policies, and what you can do when it happens. *Kaiser Health News*, October 30, 2013.
11. Radnovsky, L, Martin, TW. Cancelled policies heat up health fight. *Wall Street Journal*, October 30, 2013: A1.
12. Appleby, J. Cancelled health plans: round two. *Kaiser Health News*, October 2, 2014.
13. Brown, T. Out of network, out of luck. *New York Times*, October 15, 2013.
14. Beck, M. United Health culls doctors from plan. *Wall Street Journal*, November 16, 2013: B1.

15. Ibid # 5.
16. Cohn, J. How they did it. *New Republic,* June 10, 2010: 14, 21.
17. Greenwald, G. Industry interests are not in their twilight. *Salon*, March 20, 2010.
18. Woodward, C. FACT CHECK: Slippery claims on health law, budget. Associated Press, September 29, 2013.
19. Magge, H, Cabral, HJ, Kazis, LE et al. Prevalence and predictors of underinsurance among low-income adults. *J Gen Intern Med* 2013. doi: 10.1007/s11606-013-2354-z
20. Himmelstein, DU, Thorne, D, Warren, E et al. Medical bankruptcy in the United States: results of a national study. *Amer J Med* 122: 741-746. 2009.
21. Galewitz,P, Fleming, M. 13 states aim to limit Medicaid. *USA Today*, July 24, 2012.
22. Burke, C, 2013: the year of broken promises. December 29, 2013. http://www.newsmax.com/Newsfront/obamacare-broken-promises/2013/12/29/id/544262/
23. Condon, S. 22,000 file appeals with Obamacare site, report says. *CBS News*, February 3, 2014.
24. Pear, R. Work to bolster health website is raising cost, officials say. *New York Times*, July 31, 2014.
25. Abelson, R. Bracing for new challenges in year 2 of health care law. *New York Times,* September 2, 2014.
26. Sanger-Katz, M. HealthCare.gov still suffers from lack of transparency. *New York Times,* October 7, 2014.
27. Radnovsky, L. More health-site bugs loom. *Wall Street Journal*, November 5, 2014: A3.
28. Radnofsky, L, Armour, S. Insurance site's frailties detailed. *Wall Street Journal*, September 17, 2014: A4.
29. Caper, P. Health reforms problems run deeper than a glitch website. *Healthcare Disconnects*, December 3., 2013. htpp://www.copernicus-healthcare.org
30. Ibid # 5.
31. Wogan, JB. No cut in premiums for typical family, August 31, 2012, *PolitiFacts*, Obameter, citing Obama, B., Speech: A Politics of Conscience, June 23, 2007.
32. Ibid # 22.
33. Ibid # 22.
34. Ibid # 22.

CHAPTER 7

THE ACA: ACCESS TO CARE

Before starting this and the two chapters to follow that review the extent to which the ACA meets its original goals, five years into its implementation, let's lay out some of the key elements of the law.

The initial goal was to extend health insurance to 32 million more people by 2019, one half of that number through expansion of Medicaid. Under the ACA, uninsured people with incomes up to 138 percent of the federal poverty level (FPL) ($11,670 for individuals and $23,850 for a family of four in 2015) would be insured starting in 2014. Online health insurance exchanges would be set up for people without insurance to comparison shop for plans. Most uninsured with incomes above 138 percent of the FPL would be required to purchase insurance or face penalties; federal subsidies would be provided to help those with incomes between 138 percent and 400 percent of FPL to afford insurance. Other positive parts of the ACA concerning access included allowing parents to keep their children on their policies until age 26, setting up high-risk pools to help sicker patients get insurance, and a two-year 10 percent bonus for primary care physicians.

Table 7.1 summarizes how the ACA was intended to reform the market in terms of access, affordability and adequacy of insurance coverage. But since individual states, under the ACA, remain the main regulators of health insurance, that summary is already optimistic to the point of being doubtful. As of February 2013, just one state had approved all of these protections while only ten states and the District of Columbia had passed new legislation or issued a new regulation on at least one protection.[1]

TABLE 7.1

Seven 2014 Market Reforms Under the Affordable Care Act, Effective January 1, 2014

REFORMS	DESCRIPTION
ACCESSIBILITY	
Guaranteed issue	Requires insurers to accept every individual and employer that applies for coverage.[c]
Waiting periods	Prohibits insurers from imposing waiting periods (i.e., the period that must pass before an employee is eligible to be covered for benefits) that exceed 90 days.[a]
AFFORDABILITY	
Rating requirements	Requires insurers to vary rates based solely on four factors: family composition, geographic area, age, and tobacco use; prohibits insurers from charging an older adult in the oldest age band more than three times the rate of a younger person in the youngest rate band; prohibits insurers from charging tobacco users more than 1.5 times the rate of a non-tobacco users' rate.[b,c]
ADEQUACY	
Pre-existing condition exclusions	Prohibits insurers from imposing pre-existing condition exclusions with respect to plans or coverage.
Essential health benefits	Requires coverage of specified benefits that include 10 categories of defined benefits: ambulatory patient services; emergency services; hospitalization; maternity and newborn care; mental health and substance use disorder services, including behavioral health treatment; prescription drugs; rehabilitative and habilitative services and devices; laboratory services; preventive and wellness services and chronic disease management; and pediatric services, including oral and vision care.[b,c]
Out-of-pocket costs	Requires insurers to limit annual out-of-pocket costs, including copayments, coinsurance, and deductibles, to the level established for high-deductible health plans that qualify as health savings accounts; indexes this level to the change in the cost of health insurance after 2014.[c]
Actuarial value	Requires insurers to cover at least 60 percent of total costs under each plan; requires plans to meet one of four actuarial value tiers (bronze, silver, gold, or platinum) as a measure of how much costs are covered by the plan.[b,c]

Note: Unless otherwise noted, the provisions apply to new plans in the individual market as well as new and grandfathered plans (those in existence before the Affordable Care Act that have not made significant changes since March 23, 2010) in the small-group and large-group markets.
a Does not apply to plans in the individual market.
b Does not apply to plans in the large-group market.
c Does not apply to grandfathered plans. Note that guaranteed issue in the small-group market was already required under HIPAA and thus applies to grandfathered plans in the small-group market.

Source: Keith, K, Lucia, KW, Corlette, S. Implementing the Affordable Care Act: State action on the 2014 market reforms. The Commonwealth Fund, February 2013.
Reprinted with permission

Now, almost five years after the ACA was enacted, we can start to measure its impact on access to care. A study by the Commonwealth Fund, comparing health insurance coverage nationally before and after the ACA's first enrollment period, gives us an overview of what has been accomplished so far:

- 9.5 million fewer uninsured, with adult uninsured rate dropped from 20 percent to 15 percent.
- Uninsured rate among young adults 19 to 34 years of age fell from 28 percent to 18 percent.
- Uninsured rate for people in poverty fell from 28 percent to 17 percent in states that expanded Medicaid, but from only 38 percent to 36 percent in non-expanding states.
- 60 percent of people with new coverage saw a physician or other provider, went to a hospital, or paid for a prescription.
- Six of ten of the newly insured would not have been able to access or afford care previously.[2]

Despite this progress, however, as we look in more depth at the access problem, the scorecard is not anywhere near what we want to see, as the following section demonstrates.

WAYS THAT THE ACA FALLS FAR SHORT OF ITS ACCESS GOAL

1. States opting out of Medicaid expansion

A 2012 ruling by the U.S. Supreme Court allowed states to choose whether or not they wanted to expand their Medicaid programs under the ACA. That ruling led many red states, especially in the South and central U.S., to opt out of such expansion. As a result, more than one-half the number of people who otherwise could have been insured through expansion of Medicaid could no longer be so covered.

This outcome is ironic. Until the Supreme Court's ruling, it was assumed that all states would participate in the ACA. By January 2014, however, 24 states had not accepted federal money to expand Medicaid (100 percent federal share in the first three years, then phasing down to 90 percent by 2020). That created a "coverage gap" for 4.8 million people between the ages of 18 and 64 who weren't eligible for benefits under existing state programs and earn too little to qualify for subsidies for insurance purchased on the ACA's exchanges.

By June 2014, 22 states had accepted funding from the ACA to expand Medicaid, while 19 states had refused expansion altogether. Six states accepted ACA funding to privatize Medicaid coverage, attaching strings that don't apply to state Medicaid programs. Four states were still negotiating with the federal government over how to proceed, as shown in Table 7.2.[3]

Texas is the largest of the opt-out states, where more than 2.1 million who would have been otherwise insured will remain uninsured because of Republican Governor Rick Perry's opt-out decision. Since the federal government pays all of the costs of Medicaid expansion for the first three years, the opt-out decisions in red states are clearly political acts that put sabotaging Obama's ACA above the needs of their constituents.

States that choose not to expand Medicaid pay a big price for that political decision. In Georgia, for example, a recent study by the Urban Institute found that the state will have to spend an additional $2.5 billion over the coming decade in order to finance its share of Medicaid, while giving up $33.5 billion in federal funds that otherwise would have been available.[4]

Taking Alabama as another opt-out example, the disconnect between the goals of the ACA and its outcome in a non-expanding state is hard to believe, but unfortunately true. Low-income people with the greatest needs now get no help while better off people get federal subsidies to get insurance if between 138 percent and 400 percent of FPL. People who fall *above* states' Medicaid eligibility income levels are especially disadvantaged, as this patient's experience shows.

TABLE 7.2

States Opting In and Out of Medicaid Expansion

More than half of U.S. states are expanding health coverage for the poor either through Medicaid or an alternative model. A handful are still pursuing deals with Washington, D.C.

EXPANDING MEDICAID		
Arizona	Kentucky	North Dakota
California	Maryland	Oregon
Colorado	Massachusetts	Rhode Island
Connecticut	Minnesota	Vermont
Delaware	Nevada	Washington
District of Columbia	New Jersy	West Virginia
Hawaii	New Mexico	
Illinois	New York	
EXPANDING COVERAGE FOR THE POOR IN THEIR OWN WAY		
Arkansas	New Hampshire	Wisconsin
Iowa	Ohio	
Michigan		
NO EXPANSION		
Alabama	Maine	South Carolina
Alaska	Mississippi	South Dakota
Florida	Missouri	Texas
Georgia	Montana	Virginia
Idaho	Nebraska	Wyoming
Kansas	North Carolina	
Louisiana	Oklahoma	
NEGOTIATING		
Indiana		Tennessee
Pennsylvania		Utah

Source: Radnofsky, L.A. A National Policy on Health Care? Sort of. *Wall Street Journal*, June 9, 2014

Tanisha Fields, a 27- year-old uninsured mother of a four year-old son, has an annual income of about $7,000 with a cleaning service in Alabama. She presented to the University of Alabama's Hospital in Birmingham for treatment of a miscarriage. She earned too much to be eligible for Medicaid in Alabama, where the income ceiling is just $2,832 for a family of two, after deductions.[5]

Here are additional adverse kinds of impacts in states that have chosen not to accept federal money to expand Medicaid under the ACA:

- A recent study projects that an estimated 7,115 to 17,104 people will die among 8 million left out of coverage as a result of states' decisions to opt out of expanded Medicaid under the ACA.[6]
- More than 1 million patients who use federally funded community health centers in non-expanding states will remain uninsured, losing coverage that would have been available through Medicaid or the exchanges.[7]
- Most non-expanding states require parents to earn less than 50 percent of FPL to be eligible for Medicaid.[8]
- States developing privatized Medicaid plans seek to shift more costs onto patients by such means as expanding co-payments and setting up health savings accounts for beneficiaries without necessarily putting funds in them.[9]
- Almost 3.7 million low-income uninsured people with a serious mental illness, serious psychological distress, or a substance abuse disorder will not receive coverage under the ACA.[10]
- Almost 60,000 uninsured and low-income people with HIV/AIDS will not have coverage for care, including antiretroviral therapy, in non-expanding states.[11]

2. Narrowed networks and barriers to keeping your doctor

Accountable care organizations (ACOs) are a key element in the ACA, intended to create new payment and delivery models that theoretically could save money. They use global budgets as they organize hospitals, other facilities and providers into new arrangements that could shift from volume-oriented fee-for-service (FFS) delivery of care to a more comprehensive approach to care that includes some quality measures. Hospitals and providers in each ACO contract to provide care for an assigned patient population with the goal to provide better care at lower cost. If they succeed, they get to keep some of the savings, if quality measures are met.

In this way, the ACA has set off a new round of competition within the health care system with enlarging hospital systems and insurers playing the key roles in reorganizing providers in new ways. There are now almost 500 ACOs around the country in varying stages of development, more than half of which are for Medicare patients. CMS assigns patients to Medicare ACOs, whether they like it or not, if most of their care has been with a primary care physician participating in that ACO.[12]

ACOs raise new barriers to access for patients. Hospitals and/or insurers can change their participation in a given ACO at any time. Physicians may not know from quarter to quarter which of their patients are in their ACO because Medicare does that calculation retroactively. Insurers can change networks at a moment's notice, leaving many patients confronted with large costs for out-of-network care if they want to stay with their physician or chosen hospital.

In their quest to contract with lower-cost hospitals and physicians, insurers disrupt many patients' choices and relationships with physicians and hospitals. Hospital networks are shrinking all over the country. About 20 million people are expected to shop for plans on the new exchanges, but they will find their choices sharply limited. A recent McKinsey report found that about 60 percent of health plans available through federal and state-run exchanges include a smaller number of hospitals than comparable current health plans. Some plans limit coverage to only one or two large hospitals. In California, Santa Monica-based Consumer Watchdog has filed a lawsuit against Cigna and Blue Cross of California for misleading consumers about the size of their networks of doctors and hospitals, thereby leaving patients vulnerable to large out-of-network bills.[13]

As if we didn't learn anything from how managed care in the 1990s was discredited by decreasing choice, this is what J. Mario Molina, chief executive of Molina Healthcare Inc., says about this situation:

> *This is the grand experiment. We're going to find out what consumers value more, choice or price.*[14]

Here is how all this is playing out in Washington state for one couple shopping for a health plan on Washington's online insurance exchange:

Bev Marcus and her husband had been insured by Premera BlueCross on an individual policy that had covered most of his $150,000 in hospital bills for his heart attack and cancer care several years earlier. When they looked for a new policy with Premera Blue Cross for 2014 on the exchange, they found that none of the insurer's individual plans included any of Swedish's three hospitals in Seattle or its campus in neighboring Issaquah in its network. If they stayed with Premera, they would pay much higher costs at out-of-network hospitals, including losing their cap for total out-of-network costs.[15]

That story has become common across the country as insurers shrink their networks and compete on the basis of premiums on the exchanges. But as millions also find, skinnier networks do not assure lower premiums, they often *lose* choice on exchange offerings, and out-of-network costs can be prohibitive and potentially bankrupting.

Meanwhile, of course, a similar story is playing out for physicians. Thousands of primary care physicians and specialists have been terminated in recent months from private Medicare Advantage plans as insurers try to reduce costs and "streamline their operations," all defended by insurers as bringing "more value" to their enrollees. UnitedHealthcare, the largest plan of its kind with AARP's endorsement, plans to cut its national network of physicians by 10 percent to 15 percent by the end of 2014.[16] Many patients who gain new coverage through exchanges are encountering another problem—"phantom networks" of physicians who are incorrectly listed within networks and will not accept them for care.[17] An October 2014 study found that physician directories publicized by Medicare Advantage plans for dermatologists are very inaccurate and exaggerate actual access for patients—when contacted by researchers, only one-fourth of the total number of dermatologists listed would see new patients, and then only after a wait time of 45 days![18]

A December 2013 study by McKinsey found that more than two-thirds of health plans on the new exchanges across the country are "narrow" or "ultra narrow" in which as many as 70 percent of hospitals and other local providers are not included in network offerings. In response to a growing public backlash over these restrictions, legal protests and in some cases, legislation, are moving forward in some states.[19] HHS has proposed raising its requirement for government-run exchanges to include 30 percent of "essential community providers" (instead of the present 20 percent requirement) in their areas by 2015, but it remains to be seen how much this will remedy the current access problem.[20]

3. Primary care shortage

As more people gain insurance coverage under the ACA, many patients and families will find it difficult to find a physician, especially in primary care. According to the Association of American Medical College's Center for Workforce Studies, we have a shortage of 45,000 primary care physicians in this decade.[21] A more recent study puts that number at 52,000 by 2025.[22]

Less than 20 percent of U.S. physicians practice primary care, the critical foundation of comprehensive health care. Their numbers continue to fall as more medical graduates seek out more highly reimbursed specialties and subspecialties. This shortage further fragments health care, renders coordination of care by multiple specialists a serious challenge, and increases costs. A 2013 study found that 33 percent of U.S. primary care physicians do not accept new Medicaid patients.[23] Moreover, the original hope that the ACA would cut down on emergency room visits has not panned out, often instead *increasing* ER visits.[24]

After the first enrollment period, ending on March 31, 2014, demand for primary care has varied considerably from state to state. About 13 million people gained coverage under the ACA either through exchanges or expanded Medicaid. Primary care capacity was stressed in some states, such as Colorado and Washington State. A June 2014 report in California found that four in ten physicians listed in the State's Directory for physicians accepting Medicaid (MediCal) were either unavailable to new patients or could not be reached.[25] Additional major challenges in primary care, going forward, are the increasing stress levels, burnout, and early retirement among primary care physicians.[26]

Low reimbursement to primary care physicians has been a major barrier for them to accept care of Medicaid patients, often not covering their costs of care. The ACA attempted to ameliorate this problem by including a provision, at least temporarily, to increase that reimbursement to full Medicare rates. But a recent report found that 22 states will not continue this policy, while an additional 15 states will continue with only part of that increase.[27]

4. Delays and shortfalls in signups to the health exchanges

The original projection for signups through the ACA's new marketplaces was for about 7 million people to sign up in the first year, with about 20 million buying coverage by 2016. While 8 million were actually enrolled, enrollment was delayed, varied widely from state to state, and fell far short of expectations in many states because of glitchy website problems, difficulties with some exchanges, and the choices made by many not to sign up.[28]

The signups from the first enrollment period raised many questions, such as how many newly insured were previously uninsured, how many were in the younger age group from 18 to 34, and how many Medicaid enrollees were actually new. The answers remained cloudy, with implications for 2015 insurance rates, since the healthier, younger age groups have so much to do with where insurers set future premium rates. Only about 28 percent of signups (compared to a hoped-for 40 percent target) were in the 18 to 34 age group as insurers cautioned about future premium costs.[29] A Rand study estimated that only about one-third of sign-ups were previously uninsured, though it didn't account for the last-minute rush to enroll. That study also estimated that 14.5 million people gained coverage since the fall of 2013, while 5.2 million *lost* coverage, for a net gain of 9.3 million. The Rand researchers acknowledged that many millions had plans cancelled for not meeting the ACA's requirements, and that it wasn't clear how many switched to a new policy.[30] The gains in Medicaid coverage were also unclear, since enrollment fluctuates month to month based on income and other factors. The Urban Institute estimated the number of new Medicaid enrollees attributed to the ACA at 4.4 million.[31]

Another unanswered question, of course, is how many people will choose *not* to sign up for coverage under the ACA. Many people who visit the exchanges find coverage too skimpy or unaffordable. After the first enrollment period ending in April 2014, the CBO was estimating that about 30 million Americans will still be uninsured in 2019.[32]

Months after the first enrollment period ended, contractors were still working through discrepancies in more than two million applications to the exchanges as a major overhaul of the Healthcare.gov website was underway. An independent audit of insurance exchanges established under the ACA found widespread discrepancies in a flawed automated eligibility system, mostly involving citizenship, immigration status and income.[33] Thorny problems remained, such as devising a system to automate payments to insurers.[34] On the provider side, ACA exchange plans were an administrative nightmare, often requiring additional staff to verify patient eligibility and obtain cost-sharing and network information. Patients typically are confused about their new coverage, worried about high deductibles, and shocked by the impacts of out-of-network costs and loss of continuity of care through narrow networks.[35]

As the second enrollment period was ready to open in year two, confusion still reigned among consumers. A poll by the Kaiser Family Foundation found that nine of ten uninsured said they were unaware when open enrollment would begin, and that two thirds said they knew "only a little" or "nothing" about the exchange marketplaces.[36] A Bankrate Health Insurance Pulse survey of those who purchased policies on the 2014 exchanges found that one-half of respondents did not plan to shop again on the exchanges for 2015.[37] In a gift to insurers, the Obama administration was still not prepared to enforce transparency requirements for such things as enrollment and disenrollment data, number of claims denied, rating practices, what doctors and hospitals are in their networks, and what services are, and are not, subject to deductibles.[38] That left many millions of "shoppers" on the exchanges in the dark as to comparative costs and benefits of changing health plans.

Those who purchased coverage on the federal exchange in 2014 could automatically renew, but they would find that premiums for benchmark silver plans would cost an average of 8.4 percent higher in 2015. Auto-renewal was another perk given to the insurance industry intended to help insurers retain enrollees. If enrollees shopped for the cheapest silver plans in 2015, premium costs would go up by just 1 percent.[39] So auto-renewal is another provision in the ACA that favors insurers' markets over the needs of people seeking affordable coverage that they can depend on.

As projected by the CBO, the goals of the federal and state exchanges for 2015 are to renew all of the people who signed up in 2014 and to add about 6 million uninsured to the exchanges and 4 million to the Medicaid rolls. But many problems stand in the way of meeting those goals, including affordability of coverage, continuing website problems, wait times in a shorter enrollment period of just three months, and the challenges the uninsured face in understanding their options.

5. Dysfunctional state exchanges

The ACA provided funding to start state-run exchanges, including staffing, building and operating their websites, and marketing their offerings to consumers. State-run exchanges were expected to be financially self-sufficient beyond January 2015. Fourteen states opted to run their own exchanges, including California (the largest). The remaining 36 state exchanges are federally run. By early 2014, as the March 31 deadline approached for people to sign up or face tax penalties, state health exchanges were encountering growing problems—lower enrollments than expected, expensive fixes to glitch-ridden websites, needs for more staffing to deal with long wait times, and concerns about future solvency. Some states were considering new taxes on insurers, which would add one more factor driving insurance costs up.[40] By June of 2014, five states—Oregon, Minnesota, Massachusetts, Maryland and Nevada—were facing high expenses to fix their exchanges or switch over to the federal marketplace.[41]

Hundreds of thousands of exchange shoppers found their choices of insurers very limited. In two states—Iowa and South Dakota—a single health insurer, Wellmark Blue Cross and Blue Shield, dominate the individual insurance market and chose not to participate on the ACA exchange, both in years 1 and 2, thereby preventing consumers from purchasing subsidized coverage from the company.[42] Consumers in 515 counties, spread across 15 states, found only one available option and with it higher premiums. Insurers were avoiding areas of high unemployment with less healthy populations.[43]

6. Inadequate coverage of newly insured through exchanges

Most people signing up for health insurance on the new exchanges seek the lowest premiums for policies with low levels of coverage—either bronze or silver plans, with 60 or 70 percent actuarial value. Two-thirds of new enrollees signed up for silver plans, which brought eligibility for federal cost-sharing subsidies, not available through bronze plans.[44]

Bronze plans carry the lowest premiums, but patients with little or no liquid assets are left with 40 percent of the total costs of their health care, resulting in many foregoing essential medical care or assuming a large, potentially bankrupting debt. When patients with bronze plans seek care at community health centers, (which cannot turn them away), the centers then bill the insurers, which deny claims that fall below the deductibles. Although community health centers may try to collect means-tested payments, they are often unsuccessful, and end up having to write off the charges as uncompensated care.[45]

Many people hoping to get better coverage through gold or platinum plans are disappointed to find that they don't get extra benefits, a better network, or a more favorable drug formulary. Instead, the main difference between the metals is the amount of cost-sharing among plans.[46]

Purchasers shopping on the exchanges need to read the fine print as they comparison shop. They will find that many health care services are uncovered. Deductibles may range as high as $7,000, with copayments and coinsurance higher than expected. Networks are likely to be skinny and not include physicians or hospitals of choice. And caps under the ACA do not apply to out-of-network care.[47]

After the cancellations of policies for some 4.7 million people during the last weeks of 2013, combined with the dysfunctional government website, the Obama administration gave insurers another year to meet the ACA's requirements for individual policies. This was a sign of how worried the administration was becoming about future hikes in premiums limiting the exchanges' effectiveness to expand coverage.[48]

7. Inadequate access and coverage under Medicaid

For those qualifying for Medicaid, coverage has always varied greatly from one state to another, vulnerable to budget cuts, with no coverage for much essential care. The ACA still left Medicaid coverage extremely variable. As one example, the ACA did bring in a new requirement that most private plans, Medicare and expanded Medicaid cover the U.S. Preventive Services Task Force A- and B-rated services without cost-sharing. These services include screening for hypertension, diabetes, cancer, and depression. But a 2013 study found that Medicaid programs in many states do not cover these basic services, and that confusion reigned over what actual services would be covered in any one state.[49]

Then we have the Medicaid "coverage gap," with 5.2 million people without coverage in 24 mostly red states that did not choose to expand Medicaid under the ACA, despite availability of 100 percent federal funding for the first three years. These people, all poor uninsured adults, have incomes above Medicaid eligibility levels but below the FPL, so can qualify for neither Medicaid nor subsidies to help them purchase coverage on the health exchanges. About 60 percent of the country's uninsured working poor live in these states, prompting Dr. Jack Geiger, a founder of the community health center model, to observe:

> *The irony is that these states that are rejecting Medicaid expansion—many of them southern—are the very places where the concentration of poverty and lack of health insurance are the most acute.*[50]

This vignette puts a human face on the cruel outcomes facing patients unfortunate enough to live in states that opted out of Medicaid expansion.[51]

> *Charlene Dill was a 32-year-old mother of three who earned $11,000 a year cleaning houses and babysitting in Florida. That was too much to qualify for Medicaid and too little to afford health insurance. The ACA would have provided subsidies for health insurance if her income was more than $23,550. When she developed a heart condition, and later, abscess on her legs, she did go to emergency rooms, but couldn't afford those bills or any other care. She died of treatable conditions because Rick Scott, the multimillionaire governor with a long track record of fraud with HCA, refused to accept federal Medicaid expansion money under the ACA.*

Privatization of Medicaid programs, especially favored in red states, is another way that the value of Medicaid coverage falls short of patients' needs. Touted by proponents to be "more efficient" than public Medicaid programs, they instead extract coverage for profits. Insurers saw a new market of using new federal Medicaid dollars to expand Medicaid through the private insurance market. Arkansas and Kentucky were among the states leading this effort, which soon became known as "the private option."[52] Private managed care Medicaid programs have become common, with almost 30 million enrollees. But here is just one example of how patients lose out as profits trump coverage in a privatized Kentucky plan:

> *Because of congenital bowel problems that have required dozens of surgeries and procedures, Kaden Stone was just 3 feet 6 inches tall and 48 pounds at age 8. He relied on PediaSure, an expensive nutritional drink, for sustenance until his private Medicaid plan stopped paying for it, calling it not medically necessary.*[53]

8. Inadequate accountability for insurers

Since the ACA is built largely upon the private health insurance industry as its essential financing mechanism, the Obama administration has had to accommodate that mostly for-profit industry all along the way. This has made it difficult to contain the costs of premiums, assure competition among insurers, and maintain choice and value for consumers. Instead of accountability, we have seen insurers gravitating to the most profitable markets, avoiding unprofitable ones, and increasing their profits within an increasingly wasteful bureaucracy. Figure 7.1 shows the dramatic difference between the overhead of traditional (not privatized) Medicare and the private insurers.[54] The 4 percent figure for insurers' profits greatly understates their actual profits (which may be more than 20 percent), since it does not include return on investment of very large sums held "in trust."[55]

Affordability, adequacy and value of benefits in private plans became the Achilles heel of the ACA. In the lead-up to the bill, insurers lobbied effectively to build a number of loopholes into the final law. The ACA's requirement that insurers spend 80 to 85 percent of premium dollars on patient care, for example, was gamed by their being able to apply other costs to that number, including the costs of quality improvement initiatives, upgrades to their electronic claims systems, and most taxes and fees. Here are some other loopholes that were friendly to the insurance industry:[56]

FIGURE 7.1

Overhead of Top 5 For-Profit Insurers vs. Medicare

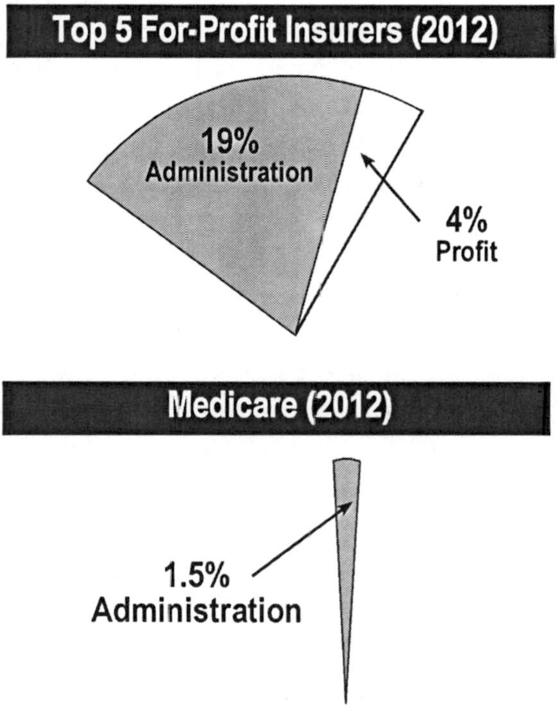

Top 5 For-Profit Insurers (2012)

19% Administration

4% Profit

Medicare (2012)

1.5% Administration

Source: Healthcare-NOW! SinglePayer Activist Guide to the Affordable Care Act. Washington, D.C., 2013, p 22.

- Self-insured employer-sponsored plans, which accounted for 61 percent of employer-based plans in 2013, were exempt from most of the ACA's requirements.
- As long as employers offer at least one plan that meets ACA's requirements, they are free to keep offering others that do not, such as very lean "fixed-indemnity" plans that pay almost nothing toward the cost of a major illness or accident.[57]
- Self-funded student health plans were exempted from annual and lifetime caps on benefits.
- Premium rate reviews, which applied only to individual and

small employer plans, were industry-friendly and lacked teeth; rate reviews are done at the state level, where they can be questioned if more than 10 percent a year, but not prevented.
- High-deductible plans and some other categories of plans were held to lower standards.
- Even after the public backlash to excessively narrow networks, the Obama administration still allows insurers to exclude 70 percent (not the previous 60 percent) of essential community providers from their networks.[58]

As could have been predicted, insurers have sought out markets that get around ACA's requirements. There is a growing movement now for private insurers to fill gaps left by the ACA and employer-sponsored plans. As deductibles increase for both employer-sponsored insurance and policies purchased on the exchanges, they see an opportunity for lower premium policies that pay fixed cash benefits for out-of-pocket costs, such as for a hospital stay or a specific disease diagnosis, such as cancer. An example of such a limited plan is one that would cost $13 to $45 per month, depending on the purchaser's age, with a cash benefit of $10,000 or $20,000 upon diagnosis of a critical illness. That would not go far in covering major new health problems, which often readily exceed $100,000 in cost. This new trend toward limited plans (now dubbed copper plans with less actuarial value than bronze plans) raises questions about the breadth of their coverage (very minimal), likely confusion among many purchasers that they have real insurance, and whether and how they will be regulated.

The trend toward supplemental coverage is reminiscent of the "Medigap coverage" that developed after the passage of Medicare in the late 1960s. Thomas Rice, a health policy professor at UCLA, states:

The early days of Medigap plans for seniors in the 1970s were marked by lax regulation, expensive policies, a lack of standards and consumer confusion . . . a policy like this has a place if it returns the vast majority of premiums in terms of benefits. If it's keeping 40 percent of the premiums, it's a disservice.[59]

9. Delays and retreats from the ACA's original requirements

In view of the complexity of the many moving parts of the ACA, it is no surprise that delays were inevitable. The website's rollout was more than difficult, as were the startups of the exchanges. As insurers and employers jockeyed for position amidst the confusion surrounding the ACA's rollout, these delays gave them some breathing room:

- April 2013—delayed enforcement from 2014 to 2015 of the ACA's cap on out-of-pocket costs of $6,350 for individuals and $12,500 for families for some employer-sponsored insurance plans.[60]
- Summer 2013—employer mandate for employers with 50-99 workers to provide coverage by 2014 was put off until 2015.
- November 2013—insurers were allowed to continue selling policies that didn't meet the ACA's requirements for at least another year.
- February 2014—employer mandate for those employers with 50-99 employees delayed another year, to 2016.
- February 2014—Companies with 100 workers or more could avoid penalties in 2015 if they offered coverage to at least 70 percent of their full-time workers (the original requirement called for 95 percent of full-time workers).
- March 2014—Plans that failed to meet ACA's requirements and were cancelled in 2013 could be continued for another two years until 2016.[61]
- April 2014—the Obama administration backed down for the second year in a row on cuts in overpayments to private Medicare Advantage plans, as called for in the ACA, instead giving them a *raise* of 0.4 percent.[62]
- The start of open-enrollment for 2015 was delayed until No-

vember 15, 2014, perhaps to take voters' minds away from the ACA during the election.

- The original penalties for not getting insurance under the ACA's individual mandate were softened by extensive use of hardship exemptions, which include inability to pay medical expenses, having had a policy cancelled, and death in the family; 23 million people were exempted from 2014 fines in this way.[63]

The hard deadline that remained in place—March 31, 2014—was the last time that people could get health insurance under the ACA without paying a penalty on their 2014 income tax.

As the delays mounted, the political free-for-all was underway as the 2014 midterm elections approached. Opponents of the ACA touted the ACA's flaws, pointing to many reasons that the ACA could not succeed and be sustainable. Supporters of the ACA counseled giving it more time as the issue of Obamacare became a major campaign issue. Meanwhile, many employers were taking a wait-and-see stance, while others were cutting workers' hours to less than the full-time requirement of 30 hours per week. Uncertainty and confusion over the ACA was widespread.

CONCLUDING COMMENTS.

Considering its bewildering complexity, it is not surprising that the ACA falls so far short of its goal to expand access to health insurance and care in the U.S. This situation is more than startup problems and raises the question whether we can justify its expense and shortfalls as so many millions of Americans remain uninsured or underinsured and so poorly covered if newly insured. We'll look more closely at costs and affordability in the next chapter.

References

1. Keith, K, Lucia, KW, Corlette, S. Implementing the Affordable Care Act: State action on the 2014 market reforms. *The Commonwealth Fund*, February 2013.
2. Collins, SR, Rasmussen, PW, Doty, MM. Gaining ground: Americans' health insurance coverage and access to care after the Affordable Care Act's first open enrollment. *The Commonwealth Fund*, July 10, 2014.
3. Radnofsky, L. A national policy on health care? Sort of. *Wall Street Journal*, June 9, 2014: A5.
4. Dispatches. GOP states refuse $423.6 billion in health coverage for poor workers. *The Progressive Populist*. September 1, 2014.
5. Weaver, C. Millions trapped in health-law coverage gap. *Wall Street Journal*, February 10, 2014: A1.
6. Dickman, S, Himmelstein, DU, McCormick, D et al. Opting out of Medicaid expansion: the health and financial impacts. *Health Affairs blog*, January 30, 2014.
7. Galewitz, P. States' Medicaid decisions leave health centers, patients in lurch. *Kaiser Health News Blog*, May 9, 2014.
8. Glied, S, Ma. S. How states stand to gain or lose by opting in or out of the Medicaid expansion, *Commonwealth Fund*, December 2013.
9. DeMillo, A. Arkansas officials eye changes to Medicaid plan. Associated Press, March 5, 2014.
10 American Mental Health Counselors Association, February 27, 2014.
11. Snider, JT, Juday, T, Romley, JA et al. Nearly 60,000 uninsured and low-income people with HIV/AIDS live in states that are not expanding Medicaid. *Health Affairs* 33 (3): 386-393. March 2014.
12. Beck, M. Hospitals give law real-world test. *Wall Street Journal*, September 27, 2013: A1.
13. Appleby, J. Consumer group sues 2 more Calif. plans over narrow networks. *Kaiser Health News*, September 25, 2014.
14. Martin, TW. Shrinking hospital networks greet health-care shoppers. *Wall Street Journal*, December 13-15, 2013: A4.
15. Landa, AS, Ostrom, CM. Many Wash. Health-exchange plans exclude top hospitals from coverage. *Kaiser Health News*, December 3, 2013.
16. Cha, AE. Doctors cut from Medicare Advantage networks struggle with what to tell patients. *Health & Science*, January 25, 2014.
17. Terhune, C. Obamacare enrollees hit snags at doctors' offices. *Los Angeles Times*, February 4, 2014.
18. Resneck, JS Jr, Quiggle, A, Liu, M et al. The accuracy of dermatology network physician directories posted by Medicare Advantage health plans in an era of narrow networks. *JAMA Dermatology*, October 29, 2014.
19. Mathews, AW, Weaver, C. Insurers face new pressure over limited doctor choice. *Wall Street Journal*, February 6, 2014: A1.

20. Wayne, A. Obamacare insurers may be forced to add medical providers. *Bloomberg Politics*, February 4, 2014.
21. AAMC. Physician shortage to worsen without increases in residency training. Washington, D.C. Association of American Medical Colleges.
22. Petterson, SM, Liaw, WR, Phillips, RL et al. Projecting U.S. primary care physician workforce needs: 2010-2025, *Ann Fam Med* 10 (6): 503-509, 2012.
23. Decker, SL. Two-thirds of primary care physicians accepted new Medicaid patients in 2011-12: A baseline to measure future acceptance rates. *Health Affairs* 32 (7): 1183-1187, 2013.
24. Tavernise, S. Emergency visits seen increasing with health law. *New York Times*, January 2, 2014.
25. Guzic, H. Directories of doctors who treat the poor are inaccurate, hurting access. *California Health Report*, June 29, 2014.
26. Shanafelt, T, Boone, DS, Tan, L et al. Burnout and satisfaction with work-life balance among U.S. physicians relative to the general U.S. population. *Arch Intern Med* 172: 1377-1385, 2012.
27. Smith, VK, Gifford, K, Ellis, E et al. Medicaid in an era of health & delivery system reform: results from a 50-state Medicaid budget survey for state fiscal years 2014 and 2015. Kaiser Family Foundation, October 14, 2014.
28. Radnovsky, L, Mathews, AW. Health plan sign-ups skew older. *Wall Street Journal*, May 2, 2014.
29. Ibid # 28.
30. Dooren, JC. Health law, economy boost insured ranks. *Wall Street Journal*, April 9, 2014: A5.
31. Radnovsky, L. How many people got Medicaid from Obamacare? It's complicated. *Washington Wire,* June 4, 2014.
32. O'Neill, S. What Obamacare? Meet 4 people choosing to remain uninsured. *Kaiser Health News*, April 25, 2014.
33. Pear, R. Eligibility for health insurance was not properly checked, audit finds. *New York Times*, July 1, 2014.
34. Ante, SE, Mathews, AW, Radnofsky, L. Overhaul of health site in the works. *Wall Street Journal*, June 6, 2014.
35. MGMA ACA Exchange Implementation Survey Report. Medical Group Management Association, May 2014.
36. Pear, R. Insurers' consumer data isn't ready for enrollees. *New York Times*, October 25, 2014.
37. MacDonald, J. Obamacare users wary of new enrollment season. Bankrate, November 3, 2014.
38. Frakt, A. Auto-renewal of health plans is a problem we don't need. *New York Times*, September 29, 2014.
39. Gorman, A, Appleby, J. Obamacare enrollment: second year an even tougher challenge. *Kaiser Health News*, October 8, 2014.
40. Associated Press. Budget model uncertain for state health exchanges. February 8, 2014.
41. Armour, S. State exchanges see costly fix. *Wall Street Journal*, June 4, 2014.
42. Bartolone, P, Capital Public Radio. A single insurer holds Obamacare fate in two states. *Kaiser Health News*, September 22, 2014.

43. Martin, TW, Weaver, C. Health options limited for many. *Wall Street Journal*, February 13, 2014.
44. Summary enrollment report. Department of Health and Human Services, Washington, D.C., May 1, 2014.
45. Daily Health Policy Report. Underinsured ACA enrollees strain community health centers. *Kaiser Health News*, September 26, 2014.
45. Gottlieb, S. In Obamacare, go for bronze health plans. For most people, buying up to gold or platinum plans is a waste of money. *The American Enterprise Institute*, January 24, 2014.
47. Lore, R, Gabel, JR, McDevitt, R et al. Choosing the "best" plan in a health insurance exchange: actuarial value tells only part of the story. *The Commonwealth Fund*, August 2012.
48. Associated Press. Administration said to ponder insurance extension. *Business*, February 6, 2014.
49. Wilensky, SE, Gray, EA. Existing Medicaid beneficiaries left off the Affordable Care Act's bandwagon. *Health Affairs* 32 (7): 1188-1195, 2013.
50. Tavernise, S, Gebeloff, R. Millions of poor are left uncovered by health law. *New York Times*, October 2, 2013.
51. Dispatches. Working mother dies of medical neglect in Florida. *The Progressive Populist*, April 15, 2014.
52. Klliff, S. Privatizing the Medicaid expansion: 'Every state will be eying this.' *Health Reform Watch*, March 8, 2013.
53. Bergal, J. Kentucky's rush into Medicaid managed care: a cautionary tale for other states. *Kaiser Health News*, July 18, 2013.
54. Healthcare-Now! *Single-Payer Activist Guide to the Affordable Care Act.* Washington, D.C., 2013, p. 22.
55. McCanne, D. Health insurers break profit records as 2.7 million Americans lose coverage. *Physicians for a National Health Program blog*, February 12, 2012.
56. Francis, T. Bare-bones plans survive through quirk in law. *Wall Street Journal*, January 16, 2014.
57. Centers for Medicare & Medicaid Services. Draft 2015 letter to issuers in the federally facilitated marketplaces. February 4, 2014.
58. Hancock, J. Insurers eye market for supplemental health coverage to fill gaps left by Obamacare, employer plans. *Kaiser Health News*, February 8, 3014.
59. Radnofsky, L, Francis, T. Health-law mandate put off again. *Wall Street Journal*, February 11, 2014: A1.
60. KHN editors. What you should know about the Obamacare delay on some out-of-pocket caps. *Kaiser Health News*, August 14, 2013.
61. Dennis, S. Administration extends Obamacare grandfathering for 2 more years. *Roll Call*, March 5, 2014.
62. Hancock, J. Obama administration retreats on private Medicare rate cuts. *Kaiser Health News*, April 8, 2014.
63. Viebeck, E. CBO: millions will dodge ObamaCare fines. *The Hill*, June 5, 2014.

CHAPTER 8

THE ACA: COSTS AND
AFFORDABILITY OF CARE

The landscape in the ACA's market-based system in 2015 is something of a Wild West gold rush among the major stakeholders. Insurers, hospitals and employers are the dominant players in determining coverage, prices and costs, each pursuing their own self-interest and financial bottom lines. Hospitals are buying up physician practices at a record clip, as physicians and medical groups lose clout in contract negotiations. Hospital systems are consolidating as they increase market share and raise prices. Insurers exclude higher cost hospitals and physicians from narrowing networks under the guise (undocumented) of quality and value for patients. Insurers are gaming the system in new ways, including restricting coverage of expensive drugs on policies offered on the exchanges.[1] Employers are shifting more costs to their employees, raising premiums, limiting coverage or dropping coverage altogether and shifting them to the exchanges.[2]

As we saw in the last chapter, oversight under the ACA is minimal. Those regulations that are enforced are friendly to hospitals, insurers and employers. The drive for profits trumps the needs of patients at every turn.

Within this environment, this chapter has four objectives: (1) to briefly examine how prices for hospital and medical services are set; (2) to assess to what extent, if at all, the ACA is containing costs for employers, for patients within the exchanges, and in Medicaid; (3) to consider whether insurance and health care are more affordable than before the ACA; and (4) to summarize the impact of the ACA to date on health care spending and costs to taxpayers.

THE PROBLEM OF UNCONTROLLED PRICES

As hospitals buy up medical groups, imaging centers, clinical laboratories, and other outpatient facilities, their prices immediately go up. Facility fees become a large part of billings as hospitals defend themselves by saying "you are paying for the walls." Anything with the name of a hospital attached costs more—a lot more. And there is no way that most of us can understand how those bills are arrived at, even if we could get copies of all the charges. The so-called charge master billing system rules and is not to be questioned or understood. A recent federal report found that prices for the 100 most common treatments and procedures vary greatly among hospitals in one part of the country to another, even within the same community. In Seattle, for example, Swedish Medical Center/Cherry Hill charges about $134,000 on average for one type of angioplasty, while the Virginia Mason Medical Center, a few blocks away, charges less than $55,000 for the same procedure.[3]

Increasingly, hospitals are being acquired by expanding hospital systems that generate higher prices, often by as much as 40 or 50 percent. Hospitals argue that their increased bargaining power gives them more leverage in negotiations with insurers and employers. But the Federal Trade Commission (FTC) has long held that these mergers and increased consolidation *reduce* competition while increasing prices. The FTC is having growing success in challenging these mergers under the century-old Clayton Antitrust Act of 1914.[4]

Prices for medical services by physicians are another black box. They vary widely from one part of the country to another and within states. As one example, the costs of obstetric care in California medical centers ranges from a low of $3,296 to $37,227 for a normal vaginal delivery while those for an uncomplicated caesarian section range from $8,312 to $70,908.[5] Other studies in California have found that charges for a routine appendectomy have ranged from $1,500 to $182,955.[6]

Overbilling by hospitals and other providers has become

epidemic as the number of diagnostic codes used in billing has grown from about 17,000 to 60,000 under the ACA. This is another example of intended efficiencies going awry, with greater complexity that only insider hospital billing personnel can understand. Gaming the system by up-coding diagnoses to increase revenue has become a new "norm" that can be better described as criminal. Pat Palmer of Virginia-based Medical Billing Advocates of America (MBAA) has just published a book, *Surviving Your Medical Bills,* that describes these brazen billing practices and helps patients to challenge them.[7]

Prices are rarely transparent for patients, many physicians dislike talking about them, and most physicians have little understanding of what their procedures and services cost; increasingly those services are billed by hospital accounting offices. A recent study of more than 500 orthopedic surgeons at seven U.S. university medical centers found that only one in five could correctly estimate the costs of the devices they implanted; their guesses ranged from about 2 percent of the actual price to almost 25 times the actual price! The lead author of that study concluded:

> *Unlike pretty much every other consumer industry, health care costs are not transparent, even for the surgeons. Each hospital system and purchasing group negotiates deals with device manufacturers and signs a non-disclosure form, promising not to share the details of those prices with anyone else. That's because medical device manufacturers strive to keep their prices confidential so that they can sell the same implant at a different price to different health care institutions.*[8,9]

Payments to U.S. physicians account for 20 percent of annual health care spending, second only to hospital services. The process whereby physicians' fees are set is ridden with self-interest on the part of competing specialties. The AMA's Relative Value Scale Update Committee (RUC) meets three times a year to recommend valuations for billing codes. Its 26 members are selected by medical and surgical specialty societies, with little representation of primary care specialties. Its recommendations are made to the Centers for Medicare and Medicaid Services (CMS), which applies them to the allocation of annual Medicare spending. The incentive among competing specialties is to maximize values of its own procedures and services. As one member of RUC describes the process:

> *Everybody sits around a table and tries to strip money away from another specialty, like 26 sharks in a tank with nothing to eat but each other.*[10]

Tom Scully, former administrator of CMS in the George W. Bush administration, is unambiguous in his assessment of the RUC process for setting physician reimbursement:

> *The idea that $100 billion in federal spending is based on fixed prices that go through an industry trade association in a process that is not open to the public is pretty wild . . . Having the AMA run the process of fixing prices for Medicare was crazy from the beginning.*[11]

As a result of this process, specialists make two to four times as much as primary care physicians and far more than specialists in other countries, where fees are typically negotiated with government payers.

As we all know so well, the prices of other health care services and products are also difficult to understand, and are consistently higher than in other advanced countries. As a result of the pharmaceutical industry's successful lobbying, the ACA prohibits the government from negotiating the prices of prescription drugs, as the Veterans Administration (VA) does so well in reducing costs to about 58 percent of what all of us pay in the private sector. It's the same story for medical devices and other products.

Insurers have considerable latitude to set prices of their policies with a generous profit. In order to attract enrollees to the exchanges, they typically compete with deceptively low premiums while increasing cost-sharing and restricting coverage in other ways. A recent survey by HealthPocket.com found that deductibles on exchange plans are 42 percent higher than employer-based policies.[12] High-deductible plans have become the norm on the exchanges, often with annual deductibles more than $5,000 for individuals and $10,000 for families.[13]

Summarizing the price problem in testimony before the Senate Finance Committee in June 2013, Steven Brill, author of an influential *Time* article in March 2013 on health care, stated:

> *Obamacare does nothing about these prices. Nothing to solve the problem—zero.*[14]

IS THE ACA CONTAINING COSTS?

This is a complicated question, since it involves costs for whom, as well as the kind of costs we're talking about. Right now, with so much attention being focused on the costs of *premiums* for insurance, it is easy to overlook the costs of *health care*, especially when it comes to out-of-pocket costs to patients.

Starting with out of pocket costs for patients and families, the story is consistent—expect to pay more all the time as unfettered market forces take hold. These three examples show how widespread this is:

- As insurers try to rein in their costs by trimming reimbursement to providers, they face a backlash from providers with new kinds of charges, such as ophthalmologists adding new "refraction fees" to assess vision acuity and emergency rooms charging an "activation fee" in addition to their facility fees.[15]
- A recent study in California found that hospital ownership of physician groups drives up costs of patient care by 10 to 20 percent.[16]
- Two-thirds of U.S. hospitals now contract out emergency care to groups of emergency medicine physicians who often opt out of insurance plans; in most states, they can bill patients for the difference between their charges and what insurers pay.[17]

As for employer-sponsored insurance (ESI), we recall that it is exempted from provisions of the ACA. Approximately 150 million Americans have some form of ESI. They can expect to pay more for their insurance for several reasons, including cuts in benefits, higher deductibles and cost-sharing, and having to pay a larger share of premiums.

Many employers will give employees a flat dollar amount and ask them to shop for their own coverage through private exchanges. Other employers will drop coverage and shift workers to state-run or federal health exchanges.[18]

Two recent studies give us clear indications of the rapid trend toward increased costs of ESI. According to a study of Fortune 500 companies, three in four companies report a rise in health insurance costs (average of 7.73 percent), having moved or planning to move employees to Consumer Directed Health Plans, and having raised or planning to raise employee contributions for health insurance.[19] A recent PricewaterhouseCoopers survey found that 44 percent of employers across all industries are considering high-deductible plans as the *only* insurance option for their employees during the next three years.[20]

Will federal subsidies be available to lower-income people with ESI? Generally, no, even when the ESI coverage falls below the ACA's standards. When employers offer their employees coverage that is considered "unaffordable" for an *individual* (not family) plan under the ACA (premiums exceeding 9.5 percent of the worker's household income), they can be eligible for federal subsidies through an exchange.[21]

With little restraint by state regulators, we are seeing premium rate hikes in both the employer-based and individual markets. Anthem Blue Cross raised premiums by up to 22 percent in 2013. The biggest factor in that increase was profits, followed by rising administrative costs (especially for marketing and claims processing), with costs of medical care only 20 percent of the hike.[22] Other rate filings in 2014 saw requested hikes up to 14.9 percent in Virginia and 26 percent in Washington State.[23] Rates for California's four largest insurers for their mid-quality standard plans in 2014 rose by at least 22 percent to as much as 88 percent in the State's Marketplace compared to their most popular plans in 2013.[24]

Premiums for 2015 will keep going up. An early analysis of medical claims by Inovalon Inc. comparing rates of serious illness in the first quarter of 2013 with 2014 found that rate to increase from 16 percent to 27 percent of claims.[25] MetroPlus, a popular new entrant and one of the least expensive on the New York exchange in 2014, has requested rate hikes of up to 28 percent in 2015 for some of its enrollees, while insurers in that state are seeking average rate increases of 13 percent in 2015.[26] In all but one of the first 10 states to file their proposed rate increases for 2015, the largest insurer in the state was seeking premium increases between 8.5 percent and 22.8 percent, with most hovering around 10 percent.[27] Florida Blue, the state's largest insurer, has announced an average rate increase of 17.8 percent for 2015.[28] Aetna's CEO Mark Bertolini expects its rate increases to be less than 20 percent for 2015 as he showed concerns over many initial enrollees dis-enrolling on a regular basis.[29]

The most expensive premiums are found in rural areas, especially where one hospital and one insurer dominate the area. These areas include Alaska, rural Nevada, most of Wyoming, parts of Wisconsin, southeastern Mississippi, southwest Georgia, and southwest Connecticut.[30]

On the individual market, uninsured people shopping on the exchanges can expect to find a wide range of premium prices, many plans with limited networks that will cost them more to have their choices of physician and hospital out-of-network, plus high deductibles, depending on the actuarial value of the plan selected. Figure 8.1 shows price points for a bronze policy, which covers 60 percent of health care costs, for a 52-year-old purchaser. Those prices pencil out to yearly premiums of $2,244 to $7,080, large sums for coverage that carries high deductibles and leaves 40 percent of health care costs up to the enrollee.[31] Deductibles are rising all the time, with a 42 percent hike from 2013 to their average of $5,081 a year in 2014.[32]

FIGURE 8.1

Price Points

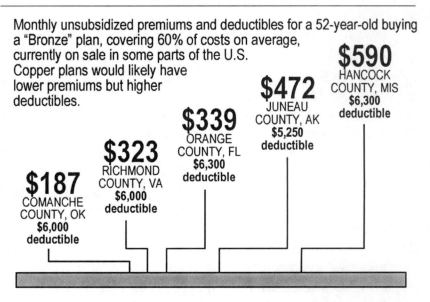

Monthly unsubsidized premiums and deductibles for a 52-year-old buying a "Bronze" plan, covering 60% of costs on average, currently on sale in some parts of the U.S. Copper plans would likely have lower premiums but higher deductibles.

$590
HANCOCK COUNTY, MIS
$6,300 deductible

$472
JUNEAU COUNTY, AK
$5,250 deductible

$339
ORANGE COUNTY, FL
$6,300 deductible

$323
RICHMOND COUNTY, VA
$6,000 deductible

$187
COMANCHE COUNTY, OK
$6,000 deductible

Source: Scism, L, Martin, TW. Deductibles fuel new worries of healthlaw sticker shock. *Wall Street Journal*, December 9, 2013.

Under the ACA, premium assistance subsidies are tied to the second lowest cost silver plan ("benchmark plan") in a given region. But benchmark status can change from year to year, and consumers have to pay the difference if they enroll in a more expensive plan. As we have already seen, insurers compete by offering skimpier network plans in order to make their premiums more attractive, and networks can change at a moment's notice. Caroline Pearson, vice president at Avalere, cautions:

Those receiving federal premium subsidies may need to switch plans in 2015 to avoid paying more than the limits established by the ACA, and the impact will be more profound for lower-income consumers.[33]

As we have seen, about 8 million people gained new insurance coverage during the first enrollment period that extended into April 2014. About 87 percent of them are eligible for premium tax credits, for which they will file with the IRS as early as January 2015. But they will face uncertainty and confusion as to the tax refunds that they will receive as well as their 2015 premiums going forward. In a recent *Health Affairs* blog, Jon Kingsdale, Executive Director of the Commonwealth Health Insurance Connector Authority in Boston, Massachusetts, and his co-author, Julia Lerche, warned us of the likelihood of refund delays and rate-shock over increasing rates—a potential one-two punch for many of these enrollees. As they explain, premium subsidy calculations are based on household income and the benchmark premium (second-lowest-cost silver plan available to each household. They point out:

> *There is a very high likelihood that the price and identity of the benchmark plan will change from year to year, as issuers adjust premiums, offer new, narrow network plans, enter new Marketplaces, and expand or contract service areas.*[34]

In states that expanded Medicaid, lower-income people will see the advantages of the ACA in gaining Medicaid coverage, but as we noted in the last chapter, eligibility and coverage varies greatly from one state to another. In the 24 non-expanding states as of January 2014, the coverage gap leaves many uninsured high and dry (Table 7.2, p. 105). Almost 5 million people in non-expanding states earn too much to be eligible for existing Medicaid programs and too little to qualify for ACA subsidies in the 138 to 400 percent range of the federal poverty level.

Some of the non-expanding states have explored or are developing privatized Medicaid programs, using federal Medicaid dollars. The CBO estimates that these programs will cost about 50 percent more than public Medicaid programs.[35] This so-called "private option" was designed as a political compromise to appeal to conservative legislators who wanted to use federal dollars to show that private markets can be more efficient than public Medicaid. But a pioneer state in privatized Medicaid has already encountered a political impasse. It seems certain that any private option program cannot survive, and that if it did, it would cut benefits to such an extent as to be unrecognizable as insurance.[36]

ARE HEALTH INSURANCE AND HEALTH CARE MORE AFFORDABLE UNDER THE ACA?

The first important point is that we need to consider both the costs of health *insurance* and the costs of health *care* in answering this question. So much attention is placed on the insurance side that it is easy to underestimate the actual costs of care. We also need to consider affordability of both in the context of other essential costs of living. Figure 8.2 shows the major costs of living for a typical family of four in 2013 in order to attain a "secure yet modest" living standard where they live, according to an analysis by the Economic Policy Institute.[37]

FIGURE 8.2

Major Costs of Living for a Family of Four*

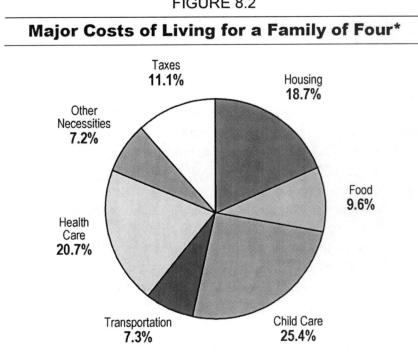

*Four-person families assume two parents and two children

Source: Gould, E, Wething, H, Sabadish, N et al. What families need to get by: the 2013 update of EPI's Family Budget Calculator. Economic Policy Institute, Washington, D.C.

The Commonwealth Fund has given us useful markers for *under*insurance: "People who are insured all year but report at least one of these three indicators: (1) medical expenses amounting to 10 percent or more of income; (2) among low-income adults below 200 percent of the FPL, medical expenses at or more than 5 percent of income; and (3) health plan deductibles at or more than 5 percent of income."[38]

Let's look at how Americans are faring in terms of affordability of insurance and health care against these benchmarks. The potential winners, of course, are previously uninsured people who get coverage on exchanges and qualify for subsidies, as well as those gaining coverage on expanded Medicaid programs. Yet, as we have already seen, there are many factors that restrict that coverage, including delayed caps on out-of-pocket costs that leave them open them to large, unaffordable health care costs.

The median household income in 2013 was $51,404, down from $55,448 in 2007 before the recession.[39] According to the Milliman Medical Index (MMI), total healthcare costs for a typical family of four with ESI in 2014 were $23,215, including payroll deductions and out-of-pocket costs. Figure 8.3 shows that the ACA has not yet changed the upward curve of health care costs. Over the ten-year period from 2004 to 2014, the MMI grew by an average of 7.6 percent per year, about three times the annual growth rate of the consumer price index (CPI) of 2.3 percent.[40]

A 2014 report from the Kaiser Family Foundation estimates that one in three Americans are having difficulty in paying their medical bills, and that most of them already have health insurance. It lists these ways that insured people may be forced into burdensome medical debt:[41]

- *In-network cost-sharing*
- *Out-of-network care*
- *Health plan coverage limits or exclusions*
- *Unaffordable premiums*
- *Other factors unrelated to insurance, including income loss due to illness.*

This report also lists these ways that the ACA does not address the underlying causes of medical debt:

- *High cost-sharing will persist under many plans.*
- *Limited protections for out-of-network care.*
- *Limits on essential health benefits standards.*
- *Lack of resources for consumer assistance.*

FIGURE 8.3

Milliman Medical Index
for a Family of Four (2014)

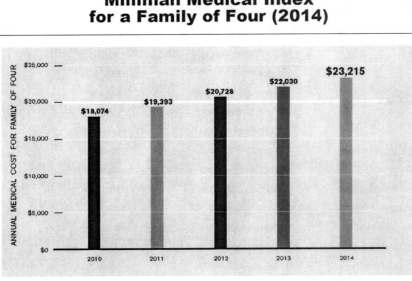

Source: Girod, CS, Mayne, LW, Weltz, SA et al. Milliman Medical Index, May 20, 2014.

Specialty drug costs give us a good example of meager coverage under an ACA silver plan, leaving patients with large out-of-pocket costs. Sixty percent of silver plan formularies place medications for such illnesses as rheumatoid arthritis, hepatitis C, HIV, cancer, multiple sclerosis, and Crohn's disease in the highest tier as specialty drugs, with cost-sharing typically in the 40 percent range. Since some of these drugs can run up to $100,000 or even more a year, they involve a financial hardship with little insurance protection.[42] The recent approval by the FDA of Merck's new drug for melanoma, Keytruda, that will cost $12,500 per monthly infusion—$150,000 for a year's treatment—gives us a new measure of how unaffordable specialty drugs are becoming.[43]

A recent analysis by Avalere Health found that people with chronic conditions are especially vulnerable to high health care costs, even when annual out-of-pocket caps kick in ($6,350 for individuals and $12,700 for families). Many chronically ill patients will spend more than 10 percent of their income (*not including premiums*, even if they qualify for subsidies on exchanges), as illustrated by this challenge facing one patient in Texas with a long-standing chronic disease:[44]

> *John Earley, an architect in Arlington, Texas, has had psoriasis for 30 years. The most effective treatment now is Humira, with twice-monthly injections costing more than $2,200. He and his wife have been in a Texas high-risk pool that has covered the drug with a $100 copayment. But since the high-risk pool will shut down within a year, John has been exploring policies on the health insurance exchange. He has found that the gold plan with the best Humira coverage would cost $20,616 a year, one-quarter of their annual income. Because other options on the exchange have high drug coinsurance charges, this appears to be his best option, even with Humira's manufacturer, AbbVie, covering most of the drug's costs through its patient assistance program.*

So how much will subsidies under the ACA help people with incomes between 138 percent and 400 percent of FPL? There are two kinds of subsidies—advanced premium tax credits and out-of-pocket assistance (aka cost-sharing reduction) subsidies. Subsidies are only available through their states' marketplace exchanges. Many factors determine the premium subsidies, which vary by income, number in the family, age, location, smoking status, and plan selected. If enrollees gain or lose income during the year, they are responsible for the difference on their year-end tax returns. To be eligible for cost-sharing subsidies, individuals or families must have incomes no more than 250 percent of FPL and have selected a silver plan. People who live in a state that has not expanded Medicaid are not eligible for subsidies if they are low-income and don't qualify for Medicaid under current rules. The Kaiser Family Foundation has produced the Kaiser ObamaCare Cost Calculator to help with this process. Table 8.1 illustrates health insurance premiums and cost-sharing subsidies for an average family of four purchasing a silver plan.[45]

TABLE 8.1

Health Insurance Premiums and Cost Sharing Under ACA For Average Family of Four for "Silver Plan"

Income% of Federal Poverty Level	Premium Cap as a Share of Income	Income $ Family of Four	Max Annual Out-of-pocket Premium	Premium Savings	Additional Cost-Sharing Subsidy
133%	3% of income	$31,900	$992	$10,345	$5,040
150%	4% of income	$33,075	$1,323	$9,918	$5,040
200%	6.3% of income	$44,100	$2,778	$8,366	$4,000
250%	8.05% of income	$55,125	$4,438	$6,597	$1,930
300%	9.5% of income	$66,150	$6,284	$4,628	$1,480
350%	9.5% of income	$77,175	$7,332	$3,512	$1,480
400%	9.5% of income	$88,200	$8,379	$2,395	$1,480

Note: In 2016, the FPL is projected to equal about $11,800 for a single person, and about $24,000 for a family of four.

Source: ObamaCare Facts: *Dispelling the Myths. Availlable at Physicians For a National Health Program*, accessed June 10, 2014

For people earning between 300 percent to 400 percent of FPL ($58, 590 to $78,120 for a family of three), the costs of getting insurance through the exchanges may be beyond their means. They may have to pay up to 9.5 percent of their income toward premiums before subsidies would apply. Those earning between 200 percent and 300 percent of FPL ($34,500 to $56,000 for a family of three) will pay up to 8 percent of their income on premiums before subsidies kick in.[46] All of these numbers are approaching financial hardship levels, *just for insurance, and not for a family's total health care costs.*

IMPACT OF THE ACA ON HEALTH CARE SPENDING AND TAXPAYER COSTS

This question cannot be answered in definitive numbers at this mid-life stage of the ACA, but the trends are not promising. The best projection at this point comes from the Office of the Actuary at CMS, which concludes that "improving economic conditions, combined with the coverage expansions in the Affordable Care Act and the aging of the population, drive faster projected growth in health spending in 2014 and beyond." That office projects that health care as a proportion of gross national product (GNP) will increase from 17.6 percent in 2014 ($17,354 per capita) to 19.3 percent in 2023 ($26,691 per capita).[47] Figure 8.4 shows enormous growth in the net costs of health insurance and government administrative costs after the passage of the ACA.[48]

FIGURE 8.4

2014 Growth Rates by Selected Sector, Before and After the Impact of the Affordable Care Act

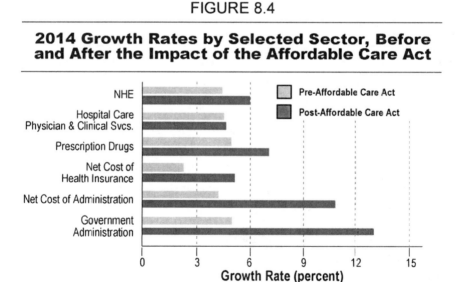

Source: Centers for Medicaid Services, Office of the Actuary, National Health Statistics Group, *Health Affairs*, October 2013.

Health care spending in the U.S. grew at the fastest pace in 10 years during the fourth quarter of 2013. This increase was driven by an $8 billion rise in hospital revenue, more than the previous four quarters combined! This was surprising in that the number of hospital days *dropped* by 1 percent in the fourth quarter.[49] A partial explanation for this is the increasing profit margin of hospital-based and affiliated emergency rooms since the advent of the ACA.[50]

As we have already seen in earlier chapters, the ACA is complex to the extreme, with opportunities throughout the private sector to game the new marketplace. At this point, it appears that none of the unproven "cost containment" strategies of the ACA, absent any price regulation, will rein in health care costs. Consolidating hospital systems and insurers are incentivized to make more money by providing less care.

A recent article sheds light on the conflicted goals of participants in ACOs as established under the ACA. The District of Columbia has just approved applications from MedStar Health, an insurer, and Johns Hopkins Medicine to build proton therapy centers that provide advanced radiation therapy that costs twice as much as standard radiation therapy but has not been shown to be more effective for most cancers. Chas Roades, chief research officer at the Advisory Board Company in Washington, D.C., which is helping to launch the MedStar insurance product, says this about the divergent goals of new profits vs. cost containment:

> *For every CEO who's considering a risk-based strategy like an ACO or bundled payments, the dilemma they have is that they have to live in two worlds at once. The ACO business isn't big enough to throw their fee-for-service revenue out the window.*"[51]

We will probably conclude several more years down the road that bundled payment systems under ACOs will be a re-run of the HMO experience that patients found against their interests.

Some insurers are forming their own ACOs, such as Blue Shield in California, which oversees 15 ACOs statewide as a competitive wedge against Kaiser Permanente, which holds the advantage of size and an integrated system of doctors and hospitals.[52] But any real savings will likely turn out to be illusory. ACOs are loosely designed managed care organizations that so far fail tests of greater efficiency and higher quality, reminiscent of the failures of HMOs in the 1990s. The several early reports by CMS are vague and fail to report how the ACOs operate, their costs vs. "savings," and the credibility of quality measures.[53] And a recent study of 145 organizations participating in the Medicare ACO programs found a substantial amount of instability of assignments of patients to ACOs, with higher-cost patients with more office visits and chronic conditions often receiving care outside of the assigned ACO.[54] Of the original 32 hospital system participants in the Pioneer Accountable Care Organization, only 19 remain in the program; the others have dropped out after failing to meet benchmark spending benchmarks.[55]

The net cost of health insurance (premiums earned minus benefits paid) applies to the private insurance industry's new enrollees through the exchanges as well as privatized government programs. Much of that increase is due to administrative costs, waste and profits. Implementation of the ACA requires a huge administrative burden for both the government and the private sector, but administration on the government side is almost five-times less expensive than on the private side ($70 billion for government administration vs. $312 billion for private in 2022).[56]

We can expect private insurers to continue their tradition of cherry-picking enrollees in new ways—trying to avoid the sick and profit from healthier enrollees. The ACA attempts to expand the number of insured and broaden the risk pool in several ways—with guaranteed issue provisions, increased coverage requirements, and taxing those who do not purchase insurance. However, there are still many ways whereby private insurers can avoid sicker enrollees and shift more costs to taxpayers. We can anticipate that as more higher-cost individuals get private insurance through the exchanges, that premiums will go up, that healthier people will not enroll or drop out due to unaffordable premiums, and that sicker enrollees will be left. This has been called the death spiral of private health insurance due to adverse selection. A recent report from the National Bureau of Economic Research describes how this is likely to play out, warning that:

The ACA's regulations may result in significant pressure to shift the cost of unhealthy individuals out of the insurance exchanges. The law would generously finance such efforts, as the federal government will reimburse more than 90 percent of the cost of its associated Medicaid expansions.[57]

Because of the many thousands of moving parts, variables, and complexity of the ACA, it is next to impossible to predict its long-term costs and outcomes. The CBO made a brave attempt to do this in April 2014, while acknowledging that "it can no longer give a reasonable estimate of the changes in the federal budget due to the implementation and perpetuation of the provisions of the Affordable Care Act." According to the CBO's latest estimates, the average federal subsidy for private health insurance premiums on the exchanges will be about $4,250 per enrollee in 2014, increasing to $7,170 per enrollee in 2024. Federal subsidies to the private health insurance industry are projected to total $1.03 trillion between 2015-2024, including $167 billion in subsidized cost-sharing.[58] That is a huge investment for such a small return to the public and taxpayers, considering that there will still be at least 31 million uninsured and that many of the "insured" will be very much underinsured.

CONCLUDING COMMENTS

As we have seen, the Patient Protection and Affordable Care Act (now shortened in everyday usage to the ACA) is a misnomer. There are too many giveaways and loopholes that favor industry, especially private insurers, to justify its name. The ACA will be very expensive, not sufficiently accountable to the public interest, and a bonanza for corporate stakeholders. Despite its good intentions, it will leave many millions of Americans uninsured and underinsured with no significant controls over prices of a largely for-profit health care industry. How can we reconcile taxpayers' costs of the ACA, with so many millions of Americans still uninsured or underinsured, and exorbitant profits on the supply side, as exemplified by Stephen Hemsley's compensation in 2012, as CEO of UnitedHealth Group, of more than $48 million?[59]

A recent plea by two oncologists, sensitized as they are to the high costs of cancer care, summarizes our current dilemma in this insightful way and calls for universal access through national health insurance:

> *With ACA now the law of the land, and its retention of the private insurance industry at the center of the health system, the trend toward high-deductible health plans, under-insurance, and cost shifting to patients will almost certainly worsen. 59 years of private sector solutions have failed. There needs to be a major paradigm shift in our approach to funding health care in the United States.*[60]

References:

1. Cha, AE. AIDS advocates say drug coverage in some marketplace plans is inadequate. *Washington Post*, December 9, 2013.
2. Francis, T. Companies prepare to pass more health costs to workers. *Wall Street Journal*, November 25, 2013: A1.
3. Ostrum, CM. Hospital prices vary wildly for common treatments. *Kaiser Health News*, June 3, 2014.
4. Pear, R. F.T.C. wary of mergers by hospitals. New York Times. September 17, 2014.
5. Rabin, RC. How much to deliver a baby? Charges vary widely by hospital. *Kaiser Health News* blog, January 16, 2014.
6. Rabin, RC. Wide variation in hospital charges for blood tests called 'irrational.' Capsules. *Kaiser Health News,* August 15, 2014.
7. Nader, R. In the Public Interest. The crime of overbilling health care. *The Progressive Populist,* October 1, 2014, p. 19.
8. Gold, J. How much does a new hip cost? Even the surgeon doesn't know. *Kaiser Health News* blog, January 6, 2014.
9. Okike, K, O'Toole, RV, Pollak, AK, et al. Survey finds few orthopedic surgeons know the cost of the devices they implant. *Health Affairs* 33 (1): 103-109, January 2014.

10. Rosenthal, E. Patients' costs skyrocket; specialists' incomes soar. *New York Times*, January 18, 2014.
11. Klepper, B. The RUC is bad medicine; it has to go, August 12, 2013. www.medscape.com
12. Ehley, B. Insurers on Obamacare: expect premium prices to soar. *Fiscal Times*, March 19, 2014.
13. Goodnough, A, Pear, R. Unable to meet the deductible or the doctor. *New York Times*, October 17, 2014.
14. Tran, A. Brill: Health law won't bring prices down for patients. *Kaiser Health News blog*, June 18, 2013.
15. Rosenthal, E. As insurers try to limit costs, providers hit patients with more separate fees. *New York Times*, October 25, 2014.
16. Terhune, C. Medical costs 20 percent higher at hospital-owned physician groups, study finds. *Los Angeles Times*, October 21, 2014.
17. Rosenthal, E. Costs can go up fast when E.R. is in network but the doctors are not. *New York Times*, September 28, 2014.
18. Appleby, J. Expect to pay more for your employer-sponsored health care next year. *Kaiser Health News,* December 20, 2013.
19. Binette, P. Survey: Fortune 500 employees can expect to pay more for health insurance. University of South Carolina, September 18, 2014.
20. PricewaterhouseCoopers. Medical cost trend behind the numbers 2015. PwC Health Research Institute, June 2014.
21. Healthcare-NOW! Single-Payer Activist Guide to the Affordable Care Act, 2013, p. 16. www.healthcare-now.org.
22. Kliff, S. Yes, Anthem Blue Cross can justify a 17 percent rate hike. *Washington Post Wonkblog*, January 8, 2013.
23. Millman, J. One health insurer wants to cut rates 6.8 percent. Another wants to hike them 26 percent. What gives? *Washington Post Wonkblog*, May 13, 2014.
24. Nirappil, F. Report: Health premiums rose significantly in 2014. Associated Press, July 29, 2014.
25. Mathews, AW, Weaver, C. Sick drawn to new coverage. *Wall Street Journal*, June 25, 2014: A1.
26. Hartocollis, A. Insurers on New York State's exchange seek significant rate increases. *New York Times,* July 2, 2014.
27. Radnofsky, L. Large health plans set to raise rates. *Wall Street Journal,* June 19, 2014: A1.
28. Galewitz, P. Florida's largest health insurer is raising exchange rates an average of 17.6 percent. *Kaiser Health News*, August 1, 2014.
29. Humer, C. Aetna says 2015 Obamacare rates increase less than 20 percent. *Reuters*, June 11, 2014.
30. Rau, J. In southwest Georgia, the Affordable Care Act is having trouble living up to its name. *Kaiser Health News*, February 3, 2014
31. Radnofsky, L. Health-law backers push skimpier insurance policies. *Wall Street Journal*, February 14, 2014.
32. Scism, L, Martin, TW. Deductibles fuel new worries of health-law sticker shock. *Wall Street Journal*, December 9, 2013.
33. Carpenter, E. Exchange plan renewals: many consumers face sizable premium increases in 2015 unless they switch plans. Avalere, June 26, 2014.

34. Kingsdale, J, Lerche, J. An ounce of prevention for the ACA's second open enrollment. *Health Affairs Blog*, August 4, 2014.
35. Ibid # 21, p.10.
36. Campoy, A, Radnofsky, L. Arkansas's Medicaid-expansion alternative stumbles. *Wall Street Journal*, February 19, 2014.
37. Gould, E, Wething, H, Sabadish, N et al. What families need to get by: The 2013 update of EPI's Family Budget Calculator. www.epi.org/resources/budget
38. Schoen, C, Doty, M, Collins, SR et al. Commonwealth Fund. Insured but not protected: How many adults are underinsured, the experiences of adults with inadequate coverage mirror those of their uninsured peers, especially among the chronically ill. *Health Affairs Web Exclusive*, June 14, 2005.
39. Plumer, B. Chart: Median household incomes have collapsed since the recession. *Workblog*, March 29, 2013.
40. Girod, CS, Mayne, LW, Weltz, SA, Hart, SK. 2014 Milliman Medical Index, May 20, 2014.
41. Pollitz, K, Cox, C, Lucia, K et al. Medical debt among people with health insurance. Kaiser Family Foundation, January 2014.
42. Gillespie, L. PhRMA, advocates: specialty drug costs for patients too high. *KHN Blog*, June 12, 2014.
43. Loftus, P. Merck's new-wave cancer drug clears FDA. *Wall Street Journal*, September 5, 2014: B1.
44. Andrews, M. Despite health law's protections, many consumers may be 'underinsured.' *Kaiser Health News*, December 31, 2013.
45. ObamaCare Facts: Dispelling the Myths. Available at obamacarefacts.com/obamacare-subsidies.php, accessed June 10, 2014.
46. Appleby, J. Some middle-class families find price of subsidized health coverage 'awfully high.' *Kaiser Health News*, February 10, 2014.
47. Sisko, AM, Keehan, SP, Cuckler, GA et al. National Health Expenditure Projections, 2013-23: Faster growth expected with expanded coverage and improving economy. *Health Affairs*, September 2014.
48. Cuckler, GA, Sisko, AM, Keehan, SP et al. National health expenditure projections, 2012-22: slow growth until coverage expands and economy improves. *Health Affairs* 32 (10): 1820-1831, October 2013.
49. Davidson, D. Health care spending growth hits 10-year high. *USA Today*, March 30, 2014.
50. Wilson, M, Cutler, D. Emergency department profits are likely to continue as the Affordable Care Act expands coverage. *Health Affairs* 33 (5): 792-799, May 2014.
51. Gold, J. Of ACOs and proton beams: why hospitals 'live in two worlds.' *Kaiser Health News Blog*, June 6, 2013.
52. Wolfson, BJ. Doctors, hospitals and insurers team up. *Orange County Register*, May 1, 2014.
53. Sullivan, K. Commentary on Quote-of-the-Day. Misleading reports on ACO savings. February 3, 2014.
54. McWilliams, JM, Chernew, ME, Dalton, JB, Landon, BE. Outpatient care patterns and organizational accountability in Medicare. *JAMA Internal Medicine*, April 21, 2014.
55. Beck, M. Health Law. A Medicare program loses 4 more providers. *Wall Street Journal*, September 26, 2014: A5.

56. Ibid # 48.
57. Clemens, J. Regulatory redistribution in the market for health insurance. National Bureau of Economic Research. Working Paper 19904, February 2014.
58. Congressional Budget Office. Insurance Coverage Provisions of the Affordable Care Act. Washington, D.C., April 2014.
59. CEO Compensation. # 8 Stephen J. Hemsley. Forbes.com, accessed February 22, 2014.
60. Drasga, RE, Einhorn, LH. Why oncologists should support single-payer national health insurance. *Journal of Oncology Practice*, January 17, 2014.

CHAPTER 9

WILL THE ACA IMPROVE
THE QUALITY OF CARE?

The third leg of the stool that best defines the structure and performance of a health care system is quality, together with access and affordable costs of care. The ACA certainly improves access to care for many people, but its impact on costs and affordability has been limited at best, as we saw in the last chapter. Now we need to look at quality of care.

The ACA has taken a number of initiatives intended to improve the quality of care. Most important, of course, are the various ways to increase insurance coverage, whether through the exchanges or expanded Medicaid. Other major initiatives include provision of preventive services without cost-sharing, payment changes encouraging quality, accountable care organizations, expanded use of electronic medical records, and establishing the Patient-Centered Outcomes Research Institute (PCORI).

The goals of this chapter are: (1) to assess the experience of the ACA in six key areas; (2) to summarize the parameters of quality of care that apply to outcomes of care; and (3) to briefly update international comparisons between the U.S. and other advanced countries in terms of quality and outcomes of care.

A MID-LIFE ASSESSMENT OF QUALITY
OF CARE UNDER THE ACA

Preventive screening

Since many patients forego mammography, colonoscopy and other screening procedures for serious illness because of costs, the ACA was well intended to include screening as a benefit without cost-sharing. But that opens the door for too much screening of people without signs or symptoms of disease with the attendant problems of false positives, anxiety over non-existent disease, over "diagnosis," and the costs and potential harms of unnecessary follow-up testing. Hospitals and providers have been incentivized to offer free screening knowing that follow-up testing will bring more revenue their way.[1]

Right off the bat, we find that profit-taking can trump evidence-based screening measures. The gold standard for efficacy of preventive procedures is the U.S. Preventive Services Task Force (USPSTF). It evaluates the most effective services and recommends against screening that lacks cost effectiveness or is likely to lead to unnecessary, perhaps harmful follow-up procedures.

Life Line Screenings is a for-profit company that advertises its services direct to *asymptomatic* consumers as "harmless," "safe," and "may save your life." It partners with hospitals and surgery centers for follow-up. Anyone can get these screenings, regardless of age, and without counseling. The company says that they have screened some 8 million people at churches, community centers, fitness centers, shopping malls, and other locations, and that about 10 percent of these screenings are positive, or "abnormal." Follow-up procedures, especially for cardiovascular findings, can be lucrative for participating hospitals, and often lead to unnecessary, expensive and potentially harmful results.[2]

Three examples of inappropriate screening tests in *asymptomatic* people are ultrasound of the coronary arteries looking for plaques or stenosis, echocardiography, and ultrasound of the heel

148

to screen for osteoporosis. Taking carotid ultrasonography, for example, the USPSTF recommends *not* screening the asymptomatic adult for carotid stenosis "because there is a moderate or high certainty that there is no net benefit or that the harms outweigh the benefits."[3] Here is the perspective of three physicians on the ethics of these commercial screening companies:

> *Because of a lack of counseling by these companies about the potential risks of an "abnormal" test result, the consumer is initially unaware that this may open a Pandora's box of referrals and additional testing to monitor or treat these abnormal findings. That most of these tests are not medically indicated in the first place is left undisclosed to the consumer, nor is there a discussion of potential adverse consequences or additional costs. . . We believe that promoting and selling non-beneficial testing violates the ethical principles of beneficence and non-maleficence.*[4]

Pay-for-performance payment system

Pay-for-performance (P4P) is an umbrella term for approaches intended to improve the quality, efficiency and value of health care. Medicare has worked with several such initiatives over the last decade. The ACA builds on this experience by establishing ACOs, a Hospital Value-Based Purchasing Program, and the Medicare Physician Quality Reporting System. Many *process* measures of performance are used, such as whether or not aspirin is given to patients with heart attacks or whether or not practice guidelines are followed for monitoring blood sugar levels in diabetic patients. *Outcome* measures are also used, such as whether or not a patient's diabetes is under control.[5]

Under the Hospital Value-Based Purchasing Program, Medicare has been giving small increases or decreases in payments to nearly 3,000 hospitals based on how patients rated their experiences and how well hospitals followed a dozen basic standards of care. But a July 2014 report found no difference in quality compared to several hundred hospitals that were exempted from the program.[6]

P4P "report cards" for physicians have been especially controversial. A 2005 survey found that only 30 percent of physicians believed that quality measures used in public reports were generally accurate. Physicians and hospitals caring for high-risk populations, such as in poor urban areas, see a higher proportion of people with more complex problems. They will tend to have lower quality scores, since socioeconomic and other factors are beyond physicians' control. No attempts are made to risk-adjust for socioeconomic factors. Risk adjustment methods are rudimentary, and invite up-coding for more reimbursement under FFS. Many physicians and some hospitals may try to avoid care of higher-risk patients to keep their quality scores up. Safety net providers and hospitals caring for poorer and disadvantaged populations are especially vulnerable to adverse impacts of P4P programs, which may actually end up *increasing* racial and ethnic disparities.[7]

Up-coding, intended to make patients look sicker than they are for billing purposes, is rampant among hospitals and physicians. Subtle changes in diagnoses can make big differences in the amounts that can be charged for services. (Table 9.1) A 2012 report by the Office of the Inspector General (OIG) of the Department of Health and Human Services found that 45 percent of chart audits at the PacifiCare unit of UnitedHealth Care "were invalid because the diagnoses were not supported."[8]

TABLE 9.1

Upcoding: The Science of Making Patients Look Sicker on Paper

No Extra Severity/Payment	Equivalent but Extra Credit
Acute kidney insufficiency ⟶	Acute renal failure
Mg. = 1.6 ⟶	Hypo-magnesemia
Delirium ⟶	Encephalopathy
Anemia 2⁰ GI Bleed ⟶	Anemia 2⁰ acute blood loss
Malnourished ⟶	Moderately malnourished
COPD exacerbation ⟶	Acute respiratory decompensation
Polysubstance abuse ⟶	Continuing polysubstance abuse

Source: Report of the Office of the Inspector General, DHHS, November 2012.

Well intended as they are, the various P4P initiatives under the ACA have not yet been shown to enhance quality, and remain controversial. Some have been rigorously studied over the last ten years, and their track record is mixed. A recent *Harvard Business Review* report drew these conclusions:

> *Overall, evidence of the effectiveness of pay-for-performance in improving health care quality is mixed, without conclusive proof that these programs either succeed or fail . . . There is little evidence that they improve patient outcomes. . . . The root [of quality problems in health care] may lie in system failures, not the failures of individual providers.*[9]

Here are some insightful observations about P4P by health policy experts:

> *An exhaustive analysis by the Cochrane Collaborative, an international group that reviews medical evidence, unearthed 'no evidence that financial incentives can improve patient outcomes.'. . . One Boston-area hospital we observed improved its quality score 40 percent just by getting doctors to change the words they wrote in patients' charts. Medicare gives hospitals more credit for saving patients with "acute respiratory decompensation" than those with "COPD exacerbations," although these terms are synonyms. That kind of practice is neither illegal nor unusual.*[10]

— Dr. Steffie Woolhandler, internist
and health policy expert

> *I do not think it's true that the way to get better doctoring and better nursing is to put money on the table in front of doctors and nurses. I think that's a fundamental misunderstanding of human motivation. I think people respond to joy and work and love and achievement and learning and appreciation and gratitude—and a sense of a job well done.*[11]

—Don Berwick, M.D., former president and CEO of
the Institute for Health Care Improvement and former
Administrator of the Centers for Medicare and Medicaid
Services (CMS)

Medicaid expansion

Some states that have expanded their Medicaid programs have demonstrated improved self-reported health status and patient outcomes as newly covered patients gain access to care. New York State has actually demonstrated decreased mortality rates. Most states, however, do not yet have good studies of outcomes, which are likely to vary considerably from state to state.

At best, Medicaid does improve access to care for those eligible, and is better than nothing. A randomized controlled trial in Oregon found that those on Medicaid did better than those without coverage. (Figure 9.1)[12] There are still major access barriers for Medicaid enrollees, however, as shown by a study comparing access to specialty care for children on Medicaid vs. private insurance.[13] (Figure 9.2) For-profit chains of urgent care centers are expanding rapidly, but most of these centers do not accept Medicaid and turn away the uninsured unless they can pay up front for care.[14]

FIGURE 9.1

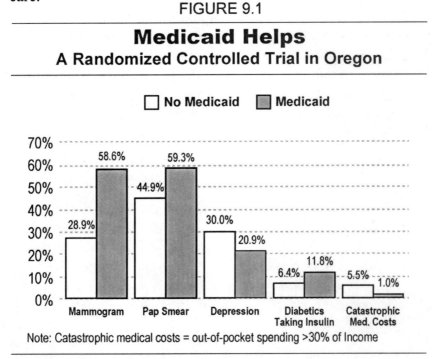

Medicaid Helps
A Randomized Controlled Trial in Oregon

☐ No Medicaid   ▦ Medicaid

- Mammogram: No Medicaid 28.9%, Medicaid 58.6%
- Pap Smear: No Medicaid 44.9%, Medicaid 59.3%
- Depression: No Medicaid 30.0%, Medicaid 20.9%
- Diabetics Taking Insulin: No Medicaid 6.4%, Medicaid 11.8%
- Catastrophic Med. Costs: No Medicaid 5.5%, Medicaid 1.0%

Note: Catastrophic medical costs = out-of-pocket spending >30% of Income

Reprinted with permission from Baicker, K, Taubman, SL, Allen, HL et al. The Oregon experiment effects of Medicaid on clinical outcomes. *N Engl J Med* 368 (18): 1713-1722,

Although new access to Medicaid in expanding states may improve quality for some, we cannot assume this to be the case, since Medicaid coverage is often so limited for many enrollees. A recent large national study that compared outcomes of the 10 most deadly cancers for patients with non-Medicaid insurance vs. Medicaid coverage, found that Medicaid patients were more likely to present with distant disease, were less likely to receive cancer-directed surgery and/or radiation therapy, and were more likely to die as a result of their disease.[15]

States that have not taken federal money under the ACA to expand their Medicaid programs will certainly experience otherwise preventable poor outcomes due to inadequate access to care. Almost 8 million Americans will not receive Medicaid in these states, and will remain uninsured. A January 2014 study foresaw these consequences for low-income adults in the non-expanding states:

> *Based on recent data from the Oregon Health Insurance Experiment[8], we predict that many low-income women will forego recommended breast and cervical cancer screening; diabetics will forego medications, and all low-income adults will face a greater likelihood of depression, catastrophic medical expenses, and death. . . . the number of deaths attributable to the lack of Medicaid expansion in opt-out states will range between 7,115 and 17,104.[16]*

Accountable care organizations (ACOs)

As we saw in the last chapter, ACOs are very much a work in progress, confusing to many, and mostly lacking in solid improvements in quality of health care. As of August 2013, about 4 million Medicare beneficiaries were in an ACO, which collectively involved more than 400 U.S. hospitals. Each ACO takes on the responsibility of caring for a population of at least 5,000 patients for at least three years. The goal is to cut costs and improve quality by improved coordination of care in and out of the hospital. Physicians and hospitals have to meet specific quality benchmarks, especially focused on prevention and care of chronic illness. Fee-

FIGURE 9.2

Many Specialists Won't See Kids With Medicaid

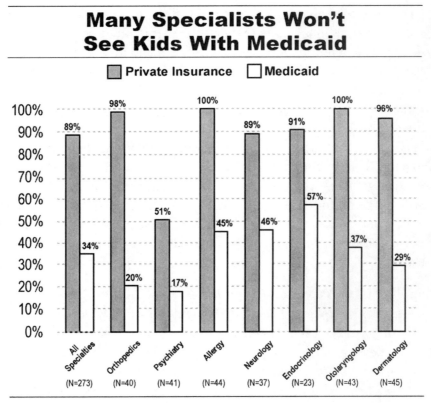

Reprinted with permission from Bisgaier, J, Rhodes, KV. Auditing access to specialty care for children with public insurance. *N Engl J Med* 364: 2324-2333, June 16, 2011.

for-service is still the main payment method, and physicians may earn a bonus if they meet quality benchmarks. Patients don't pick their ACO, and may not even be aware that they are in one. They are free to see physicians outside of an ACO.[17]

In its 2012 performance report on 141 Medicare ACOs, CMS used just five quality measures, including four assessing care of diabetes. Twenty-eight other measures that had originally been selected were not reported, as they were considered out of date, not easily understood, or otherwise not useful.[18]

Electronic health records (EHRs)

The federal government has used financial incentives to move physicians and other providers away from paper records to EHRs in an effort to improve efficiency and coordination of care. Here again, this is no panacea for quality improvement. We have an expanding health information technology (HIT) industry with many competing systems that don't necessary talk to each other. Epic, the country's leading EHR system in terms of market share, is based just outside of Madison, Wisconsin. Epic systems are "customized" for each of the three hospitals in Madison so that they don't directly communicate with each other and physicians have a learning curve to deal with each one.

A February 2014 report found that two-thirds of physicians who adopted EHRs would not purchase their system again because of poor functionality and high costs. EHRs change the physician-patient interaction in a given visit, with the physician necessarily focusing more on the computer screen than looking at or listening to the patient. Almost one-half of physicians felt that patient care was worse after going to that system.[19]

It was initially assumed by many that wider adoption of electronic health records by physicians and hospitals would improve efficiency and patient safety, reduce diagnostic testing, and save money. That assumption has been debunked by a number of national studies. One study showed that physicians' access to electronic access for test results does not reduce the ordering of unnecessary tests.[20] Another found that electronic health records facilitate the up-coding of tests performed, and that many hospitals thereby *raise* their emergency department billings to Medicare.[21] Other studies have found that less than one-half of the nation's hospitals can transmit a patient care document and that only 14 percent of physicians can exchange patient data with outside hospitals or other providers. [22]

Cybercrime poses an additional and growing threat, in spite of the privacy and security protections of the Health Insurance Portability and Accountability Act (HIPAA). A recent study has found that some 94 percent of health care institutions have been victims of cyberattacks. These involved data loss, monetary theft, attacks on medical devices, or attacks on infrastructure.[23]

The Patient-Centered Outcomes Research Institute (PCORI)

An important component of the ACA was the establishment in 2010 of PCORI to oversee and set guidelines for urgently needed comparative effectiveness research. Recall from earlier chapters that up to one-third of health care services provided in the U.S. are inappropriate or unnecessary, with some potentially harmful. We should certainly be able to expect that health care services that are delivered are efficacious and cost-effective in terms of value. But PCORI is another example of a good intention rendered ineffective by political realities.

PCORI was hobbled from the start by the ACA's specific bans on its authority to dictate coverage and reimbursement policies, or to set clinical guidelines for federal health programs. Its recommendations could go nowhere without buy-in from such stakeholders as the medical community and the drug and medical device industries. Although PCORI was well funded by the ACA, the legislation included a "sunset date" of September 2019, a limited period to persuade Congress to re-authorize funding for the institute.[24]

As we have seen, many stakeholders on the supply side of the delivery system profit from marketing and providing tests, procedures and services of doubtful cost-effectiveness. As long as the business culture of medicine continues, PCORI faces an uphill battle for legitimacy, influence, and viability.

Examples of the need for an institute such as PCORI are everywhere, as these examples suggest:

- Brachytherapy, a newer type of radiation therapy for breast cancer, is shorter than standard treatment, costs twice as much, and has not yet been shown to be cost-effective; a recent national study found that it is being provided at for-profit hospitals more than at not-for-profits.[25]
- About 90 percent of all new drugs approved by the FDA are no more effective than existing drugs.[26]

- The number of defective Class 1 recalls of medical devices—those which carry a significant probability of death—increased from 7 in 2003 to 57 in 2012.[27]
- The FDA has approved testosterone drugs only for men with hypogonadism and low testosterone levels; a randomized study funded by the NIH has shown a fivefold increase in adverse cardiovascular events in men taking these drugs, including heart attacks and strokes; another landmark study from 27 randomized clinical trials over the last 30 years found an increase of more than 50 percent in these adverse events; yet "research" conducted by the drug industry of their own products has found no increased cardiovascular risk, the drug industry actively promotes them, and one in four men taking these drugs has not had blood tests confirming "low T."[28]

PARAMETERS OF QUALITY OF CARE

Quality of care is difficult to measure meaningfully because of the breadth of issues raised in its definition and measurement. For starters, access, costs and quality are closely intertwined—there can be *no* quality of care without access to essential services. If we think more broadly about quality, we can see how the few measures in use today miss the target.

In its 2001 report, *Crossing the Quality Chasm: A New System for the 21ˢᵗ Century,* the Institute of Medicine identified these key dimensions of quality of care:[29]

1. *Safe*—avoiding injuries to patients from the care that is intended to help them.
2. *Effective*—providing services based on scientific knowledge to all who could benefit and refraining from providing services to those not likely to benefit (avoiding underuse and overuse, respectively).
3. *Patient-centered*—providing care that is respectful of and responsive to individual patient preferences, needs, and values and ensuring that patient values guide all clinical decisions.

4. *Timely*—reducing waits and sometimes harmful delays for both those who receive and those who give care.

There are many important subtleties that determine how useful any quality measures can be. As one example, inappropriate or unnecessary care, even if provided with high technical competence, is still poor care. As another, some health outcomes, such as improvements in laboratory tests, have little or nothing to do with what matters to patients, such as quality of life, morbidity or mortality. Still another example relates to whether care is delivered by for-profit health plans or not-for-profit ones—publicly traded, investor-owned, for-profit Medicaid health plans have been shown to spend less on patient care and have worse quality of care compared to their not-for-profit counterparts.[30]

INTERNATIONAL COMPARISONS OF QUALITY OF CARE

The U.S. has been an outlier for many years in having the most expensive system in the world, together with restricted access and worse outcomes of care. The Commonwealth Fund has compared access, affordability and outcomes of care in the U.S. with other advanced countries over many years. Its 2014 report comparing the U.S. with six other countries in quality, access, efficiency and equity of care, as well as long, healthy productive lives and health expenditures per capita, is summarized in Figure 9.3— a poor report card for the U.S. across the board.[31]

In its latest report comparing the U.S. with ten other advanced countries, the Commonwealth Fund found no significant change in these comparisons. Its 2013 report showed that, among U.S. adults:

- 37 percent did not see a doctor when sick, did not get recommended care, or failed to fill a prescription because of cost, compared with 4 percent in the U.K. and 6 percent in Sweden.
- 23 percent had serious problems paying medical bills or were unable to pay them, compared with 13 percent in France and

6 percent or less in the U.K., Sweden and Norway.

- 41 percent spent $1,000 or more out-of-pocket for care in the past year—the highest rate of any country surveyed.
- 75 percent said their health care system "needs to undergo fundamental changes or be rebuilt completely."[32]

FIGURE 9.3

Overall Ranking of Eleven Health Care Systems

COUNTRY RANKINGS	AUS	CAN	FRA	GER	NETH	NZ	NOR	SWE	SWIZ	UK	US
OVERALL RANKING (2013)	4	10	9	5	5	7	7	3	2	1	11
Quality Care	2	9	8	7	5	4	11	10	3	1	5
Effective Care	4	7	9	6	5	2	11	10	8	1	3
Safe Care	3	10	2	6	7	9	11	5	4	1	6
Coordinated Care	4	8	5	10	5	2	7	11	3	1	6
Patient-Centered Care	5	8	10	7	3	6	11	9	2	1	4
Access	8	9	11	2	4	7	6	4	2	1	9
Cost-Related Problem	9	5	10	4	8	6	3	1	7	1	11
Timeliness of Care	6	11	10	4	2	7	8	9	1	3	5
Efficiency	4	10	8	9	7	3	4	2	6	1	11
Equity	5	9	7	4	8	10	6	1	2	2	11
Healthy Lives	4	8	1	7	5	9	6	2	3	10	11
Health Expenditures/Capita, 2011**	$3,800	$4,522	$4,118	$4,495	$5,099	$3,182	$5,669	$3,925	$5,643	$3,405	$8,508

Notes: *Includes ties, **Expenditures shown in $US PPP (Purchasing Power Parity). Australian $ data from 2010.

Source: Reprinted with permission from Davis, K, Stremikis, K, Squires, D et al. *Mirror, Mirror on the Wall, 2014 Update: How the U.S. Health Care System Compares Internationally.* The Commonwealth Fund, June 16, 2014.

CONCLUDING COMMENT

The more we try to increase access, contain costs, and improve quality of care with incremental tweaks to our dysfunctional multi-payer system, the more complicated it all gets without real improvement. Twenty years of these tweaks have fallen far short of the need.

These ten principles were advanced in a 1994 paper explaining how a universal, single-payer national health program is key to improving quality in our health care delivery system:[33]

1. *There is a profound and inseparable relationship between access and quality: universal insurance coverage is a prerequisite for quality care.*
2. *The best guarantor of universal high-quality care is a unified system that does not treat patients differently based on employment, financial status, or source of payment.*
3. *Continuity of primary care is needed to overcome fragmentation and overspecialization among health care practitioners and institutions.*
4. *A standardized confidential electronic medical record and resulting database are key to supporting clinical practice and creating the information infrastructure needed to improve care overall.*
5. *Health care delivery must be guided by the precepts of continuous quality improvement (CQI).*
6. *New forums for enhanced public accountability are needed to improve clinical quality, to address and prevent malpractice, and to engage practitioners in partnerships with their peers and patients to guide and evaluate care.*
7. *Financial neutrality for medical decision making is essential to reconcile distorting influences of physician payment mechanisms with ubiquitous uncertainties in clinical medicine.*
8. *Emphasis should shift from micromanagement of providers' practices to macroallocation decisions. Public control over expenditures can improve quality by promoting regionalization, coordination, and prevention.*
9. *Quality required prevention. Prevention means looking beyond medical treatment of sick individuals to community-based public health efforts to prevent disease, improve functioning and well-being, and reduce health disparities.*
10. *Affordability is a quality issue. Effective cost control is needed to ensure availability of quality health care both to individuals and the nation.*

These principles are timeless, apply fully today, and give us a way out of our troubles. Can we learn, and will we ever learn from our incremental failures?

References

1. Welch, HG. The problem with free health care. *New York Times*, April 30, 2014.
2. Gold, J. Prevention for profit: questions raised about some health screenings. *Kaiser Health News*, October 28, 2013.
3. U.S Preventive Services Task Force. Screening for carotid artery stenosis: U.S. Preventive Services Task recommendation statement. *Ann Intern Med* 147: 854-859, 2007.
4. Wallace, EA, Schuman, JH, Weinberger, SE. Ethics of commercial screening tests. *Ann Intern Med* 157 (10): 747-748, 2012.
5. Health Policy Brief: Pay-for-Performance. *Health Affairs*, October 11, 2012.
6. Rau, J. First look at Medicare quality incentive program finds little benefit. *Kaiser Health News Blog*, August 6, 2014.
7. Health Policy Brief. Public Reporting on Quality and Costs. *Health Affairs*, March 8, 2012.
8. Report of the Office of the Inspector General, DHHS, November 2012.
9. Ryan, AM, Werner, RM. Doubts about pay-for-performance in health care. *HBR Blog Network*, October 9, 2013.
10. Woolhandler, S. Should physician pay be tied to performance? No, the system is too easy to game—and too hard to set up. *Wall Street Journal*, June 16, 2013.
11. Berwick, D. as quoted in Galvin, R. Interview. 'A deficiency of will and ambition'. *Health Affairs Web Exclusive* W 5-5, January 12, 2005.
12. Baicker, K, Taubman, SL, Allen, HL et al. The Oregon Experiment—effects of Medicaid on clinical outcomes. *N Engl J Med* 368 (18(: 1713-1722, May 2, 2013.
13. Bisgaier, J, Rhodes, KV. Auditing access to specialty care for children with public insurance. *N Engl J Med* 364: 2324-2333, June 16, 2011.
14. Creswell, J. Race is on to profit from rise of urgent care. *New York Times*, July 9, 2014.
15. Walker, GV, Grant, SR, Guadagnolo, A et al. Disparities in stage at diagnosis, treatment, and survival in nonelderly adult patients with cancer according to insurance status. Journal of Clinical Oncology, August 4, 2014.
16. Dickman, S, Himmelstein, Du, McCormick, D et al. Opting out of Medicaid expansion: The health and financial impacts. *Health Affairs Blog*, January 30, 2014.
17. Gold, J. FAQ on ACOs: Accountable Care Organizations, explained. *Kaiser Health News*, August 23, 2013.
18. Rau, J. Medicare data show wide differences in ACOs patient care. *Kaiser Health News*. February 21, 2014.

19. Verdon, DR. Physician outcry on EHR functionality, cost will shake the health information technology sector. *Medical Economics*, February 10, 2014.
20. McCormick, D, Bor, DH, Woolhandler, S et al. Giving office-based physicians electronic access to patients' prior imaging and lab results did not deter ordering of tests. *Health Affairs* 31 (3): 488-495, March 2012.
21. Abelson, R, Creswell, J, Palmer, G. Medicare bills rise as records turn electronic. *New York Times*, September 21, 2012.
22. Creswell, J. Doctors hit a snag in the rush to connect. *New York Times*, September 30, 2014.
23. Perakslis, ED. Cybersecurity in health care. *N Engl J Med* 371(5): 395-397, July 31, 2014.
24. Dayoub, E. Lessons from abroad and at home: how PCORI can improve quality of care (and prove it) by 2019. *Health Affairs Blog,* May 2, 2014.
25. Rabin, RC. Study: costly breast cancer treatment more common at for-profit hospitals. *KHN Blog*, April 28, 2014.
26. Light, DW. Risky drugs: why the FDA cannot be trusted. The Lab @ Edmond J. Safra Center for Ethics, Harvard University. Available at http:://www.ethics.harvard.edu/lab/blog/312-risky-drugs
27. Burton, TM. Recalls doubled of medical devices. *Wall Street Journal*, March 21, 2014: B4.
28. Ryan, A. Empty promises from dangerous testosterone-containing drugs. *Public Citizen News,* March/April 2014, p. 6.
29. Institute of Medicine. Committee on Quality of Health Care in America. *Crossing the Quality Chasm: A New Health System for the 21st Century*. Washington, D.C., 2001.
30. McCue, MJ, Bailit, MH. Assessing the financial health of Medicaid managed care plans and the quality of patient care they provide. New York. *The Commonwealth Fund*, June 15, 2011.
31. Davis, K, Stremikis, K, Squires, D, Schoen, C. *Mirror, Mirror on the Wall*, 2014 Update: How the U.S. Health Care System Compares Internationally. *The Commonwealth Fund*, June 16, 2014.
32. Schoen, C, Osborn, R, Squires, D et al. Access, affordability, and insurance complexity are often worse in the United States compared to 10 other countries. *Health Affairs Web Exclusive*, November 14, 2013.
33. Schiff, G, GD, Bindman, AB, Brennan, TA, et al. A better quality alternative: single-payer national health system reform. *JAMA* 272: 803-808, 1994.

CHAPTER 10

LESSONS FROM THE ACA'S FAILURES

Those who cannot remember the past are condemned to repeat it. —George Santayana

Five years into the implementation of the Affordable Care Act, about midway in its original legislative life 2010-2019, what can we say about its future, and what have we already learned from these initial years? The last four chapters have discussed the ACA's promises vs. realities, as well its initial impacts on access, costs, affordability, and quality of care. Many will say that it is too early to assess its ultimate outcome, but my position is that the first five years' experience has already set in place the trends and that we can now see where the ACA is going—too far short of the reforms urgently needed.

This chapter has two goals: (1) to briefly summarize the ACA at mid-life based on our findings of the foregoing chapters; and (2) to put forward 10 lessons we can already learn from its startup.

THE ACA AT MIDLIFE

Despite the relentless claims by the right that the ACA, or Obamacare, is a government takeover, the opposite is true. It was crafted by private interests and enabled by a government seeking to redirect private markets in the public interest.

Tom Scully, former administrator of the Centers for Medicare and Medicaid Services (CMS) during the George W. Bush administration, was the keynote speaker in October 2013 at a meeting of the Potomac Research Group, a Beltway firm that advises large investors on government policy. He got it right in this assessment of the ACA:

> *Obamacare is not a government takeover of medicine. It is the privatization of health care. . . It's going to make some people very rich.*[1]

In his 2014 book, *Mother of Invention: How the Government Created "Free-Market" Health Care,* Robert Field, professor of law and of health policy and management at Drexel University, agreed with that assessment:

> *Obama's health reform plan is a true public-private partnership in the mold of a longstanding American paradigm. The government created a new regulatory infrastructure within which private health care finance can function. It contributes considerable financial support, estimated at more than $1 trillion over the first 10 years, to subsidize the public's use of the new finance mechanisms. Built on this new foundation, private companies can sell products to a vastly expanded customer base.*[2]

To be fair, the ACA has accomplished some good things for many Americans, including these examples:

- Providing for parents to keep their children on their policies until age 26
- Prohibiting exclusions based on pre-existing conditions and banning of annual and lifetime limits
- Establishing government-sponsored exchanges in every state whereby uninsured people can shop for coverage
- 57 percent of the 7 million people enrolling on the exchanges during the first enrollment period were previously uninsured, with seven out of ten uninsured for two years or more.[3]
- About 7 million people have gained new Medicaid coverage and another 4-plus million have received government subsidies to buy insurance policies on the new exchanges

- Nationally, the uninsured rate peaked at 18 percent in the third quarter of 2013, then dropped to 13.4 percent in the second quarter of 2014.[4]
- Providing some new funding for community health centers
- Providing for some increased reimbursement of primary care physicians on a temporary basis

Following, however, are some of the facts on the ground of the ACA at age 5 that represent ongoing problems:

- Many employers are shifting from defined benefit to a defined contribution system of just paying a certain amount toward their employees' coverage; many others are dropping coverage or shifting employees to the new exchanges, relieving themselves of their growing burden of coverage.
- Although 8 million people have signed up for coverage on the exchanges, it appears that many millions will shy away from them.
- Thousands of people signed up on the exchanges, paid their premiums, then found that they were not insured; three months after the first enrollment period ended, Minnesota had a backlog of some 6,500 requests for changes due to a life event, such as getting married or having a baby, that requires coverage to be updated.[5]
- The individual mandate has been weakened by the expansion of hardship exemptions to the point that almost 90 percent of the nation's 30 million uninsured will not pay a penalty for not buying health insurance.[6]
- Insurers are raising premiums with little restraint and offering policies of decreasing value, including many bare-bones policies not deserving of the word "insurance."
- Narrow networks are limiting choice of hospital and physician across the country as expanding hospital systems gain near-monopoly market shares.
- The shortage of primary care physicians limits access for many millions of newly "insured" patients, especially those on Medicaid with low reimbursement rates.

- There is no evidence yet that quality of care has been significantly improved by the ACA.
- The administrative bureaucracy required to implement the ACA has increased exponentially, especially on the private side.
- As new profitable markets emerge, we have entered a new era of profiteering without adequate government oversight.
- From the beginning, we knew that 31 million Americans would remain uninsured in 2019 after full implementation of the ACA; to that number we need to add an unknown number of people who decide not to sign up for insurance through the exchanges or find it unaffordable; in addition, the pending ruling by the U.S. Supreme Court, expected in June or July of 2015, will make coverage unaffordable for many Americans if it rules against subsidies and tax credits under the ACA. In that case, we may end up with a number of uninsured in 2024 not too far short of the uninsured before the ACA.
- Public support for the ACA remains mixed, with nearly one-half of Americans supportive (especially those who have received new coverage and tax credits) and the other almost one-half unfavorable, especially younger adults and those who had prior coverage but had to switch because of cancellations or their plans not meeting the ACA's requirements.[7]

TEN LESSONS—ALL PREDICTABLE AND REAL

1. Health care "reform" through the ACA was framed and hijacked by corporate stakeholders, themselves in large part responsible for system problems of health care and dedicated to perpetuating their self-interests in an unfettered health care marketplace.

The opening assumption by framers across the political spectrum was that we had to build on the existing market-based system. The interests of insurers, the drug and medical device industries, hospitals and organized medicine took precedence over the needs of patients for broad access to affordable quality health care. Although deregulated markets were largely responsible for system problems of access, costs and quality for many years, the architects of the ACA were not willing to confront corporate stakeholders in the status quo where the business "ethic" prevails.

More fundamental questions, such as whether health care is a right or a privilege based on ability to pay, whether health care is just a commodity for sale on an open market, or whether universal access to care is the overriding goal, were not raised during the debate leading up to the passage of the ACA. Instead, the right argued that markets would fix our problems (as they had supposedly done for more than 25 years). The left focused on details that the public found difficult to understand—ranging from exchanges to triggers—but remaining silent on the bigger policy questions.

The political process was commandeered by corporate money, which bought most of the media coverage and many legislators on both sides of the aisle. Drafters of the legislation often had major unreported conflicts of interest, as exemplified by Elizabeth Fowler, the lead author of the Senate Finance Committee's bill, who had served as vice president for public policy at Wellpoint, the country's largest insurer.[8] Senator Max Baucus, chairman of the pivotal Senate Finance Committee, further illustrates how money controlled the political process. As we saw in Chapter 5, he took in the largest campaign contributions of any senator from the health sector in 2008—more than $1.1 million in 2008 and almost $2.8 million over his career.[9] Lobbyists also played a major role in getting the ACA passed in its final form. By the time of its enactment, some 1,750 organizations and businesses had hired about 4,525 lobbyists, eight for every member of Congress, at a cost of $1.2 billion.[10]

Lest we think that influence peddling by lobbyists is less of a problem since "tightening up" in 2007 of the Lobbying Disclosure Act (LDA) of 1995, think again. Most lobbying today is carried out under the radar by unregistered influence peddlers who exploit the loopholes of the LDA, which is also minimally enforced. James Thurber, an adviser to the American Bar Association's lobbying reform task force, estimates that the number of working lobbyists, most unregistered, is in the range of 100,000. A November 2013 report from McKinsey & Company put the "business value at stake from government and regulatory intervention" at about 30 percent of earnings for companies in most sectors—in other words, what is spent on lobbying brings far more revenue than the cost of lobbying.[11]

2. **You can't contain health care costs by leaving for-profit health care industries to pursue their business "ethic" in a deregulated marketplace.**

With friendly federal subsidies, new markets through health care exchanges and expansion of Medicaid, and no effective price controls, corporate stakeholders on the supply side are whistling on their way to the bank. One venture capitalist promoting investment opportunities for private exchanges under the ACA sees the likelihood "to turn chaos into gold: while much of the U.S. populace sees chaos as they watch Obamacare unfold, the investment community sees opportunity to prosper."[12] Indeed, healthcare stocks climbed by almost 40 percent in 2013, the highest of any sector in the S&P 500.[13] Venture capital funding for health technology firms soared by 176 percent in the first eight months of 2014 compared to the previous year.[14]

We are seeing increasing numbers of mergers, or attempted mergers, of health care corporations seeking an overseas address as a means to lower their corporate tax rates. The so-called "tax-inversion" frenzy in the pharmaceutical industry has led to growing regulatory concerns and the need to overhaul our business tax system.[15] The same pattern is unfolding in the medical device industry, as illustrated by Medtronic Inc.'s recent purchase of its Ireland-based rival, Covidien PLC, for $42.9 billion.[16]

We have known for years that health care markets do not operate the same way as other markets. As an example, a nine-year Community Tracking Study of 12 major U.S. health care markets found four barriers to efficiency and quality of care: (1) providers' market power; (2) absence of efficient provider systems; (3) employers' inability to push the system toward efficiency and quality; and (4) insufficient health care competition.[17]

Since the passage of the ACA, there has been a modest, probably temporary slowdown in health care spending as part of the recession and increased cost-sharing for consumers. However, prices and costs continue to escalate for hospitals, physicians, drug and medical device manufacturers, and other members of the medical-industrial complex. Increasing consolidation has taken place among hospital systems and providers, gaining near monopoly market shares in many parts of the country.

3. You can't reform the delivery system without reforming the financing system.

As with the failed Clinton health plan and other reform attempts before it, the ACA built upon our present largely for-profit multi-payer financing system. In seeking to cover more people at more affordable costs, it was focused on trying to change the delivery system—a naive and ill-informed strategy.

In the aftermath of the ACA, the private health insurance industry has become even more complex and intrusive than before as it profits from new subsidized markets. We will learn that we have to change the *financing* system if we are to have any hope of changing the *delivery* system and contain health care costs.

In his 2013 *Health Care Disconnects* blog, Dr. Samuel Metz notes three characteristics of successful financing systems in every other industrialized country:

1. universal access to comprehensive care without discrimination against the sick, poor, or unemployed;
2. encouragement of patients to seek health care without financial penalty; and
3. financing by publicly accountable, transparent, not-for-profit agencies.

Instead we have insurers trying to avoid costlier, sicker patients and gaming the system in other ways to maximize their profits and keep their shareholders happy. Dr. Metz's advice:

1. *If you want comprehensive care for more people for less money, reform the financing system.*
2. *If you want a dramatic reduction in costs without compromising quality, reform the delivery system.*
3. *If you want Rule #2 to work, you must first apply Rule #1.*[18]

4. The private health insurance industry does not offer enough value to be bailed out by government.

The private health insurance industry has had a long run since shifting to medical underwriting in the early 1960s and a mostly for-profit status. As the costs and prices of health care have spiraled upward for more than the last three decades, it finds itself increasingly dependent on the government for its very existence. Its many perks from the government include tax exemptions for employer-sponsored insurance; privatized Medicare and Medicaid programs, including long-standing overpayments to Medicare Advantage plans; and more recently, friendly provisions in the ACA, such as subsidized premiums through the exchanges, expansion of Medicaid, and a "risk corridor system" to protect insurers from losses in the new marketplace. The latest gift from the Obama administration to the insurance industry is allowing insurers to self-renew automatically for 2015 for plans obtained through the ACA's exchanges in the first enrollment period; critics have questioned whether insurers will be tempted to raise premiums since consumers will be less likely to leave a plan that has been renewed.[19]

After a 15-year history with private Medicaid managed care organizations, Connecticut, the "insurance capitol of the world", will take over its Medicaid program for more than 400,000 children and parents. Private insurers, including Aetna, never demonstrated that they could provide lower costs and better care, as they claimed.[20] We can expect that privatized Medicaid programs in other states will cost more and deliver less value as they pursue their business models.

Here are some of the major reasons why private insurers warrant no bailout by government at taxpayer expense, with examples:

• *Continued discrimination against the sick*

A recent letter from more than 300 patient advocacy groups to the Secretary of Health and Human Services detailed ongoing ways that insurers, despite the supposed consumer protections of the ACA, continue to discriminate against the sick, including benefit designs that limit access, restrictive drug formularies, inadequate provider networks, high cost-sharing, and deceptive marketing practices with a lack of plan transparency.[21]

• *Fragmentation, inefficiency and high administrative overhead*

The administrative overhead of the 1,300 private insurers in the U.S. is more than five times higher than that of the single-payer program in two Canadian provinces,[22] while the overhead of private Medicare Advantage plans averages 19 percent vs. 1.5 percent for traditional Medicare.[23]

• *Increasing epidemic of underinsurance*

More than 1 million families seek bankruptcy protection each year, two-thirds because of medical bills; 60 percent of them *had* private coverage at the onset of their bankrupting illness or accident[24]; the insurance industry is now lobbying for so-called copper plans with an actuarial value of only 50 percent, which would make underinsurance even more widespread[25]; about 40 percent of people gaining coverage through the ACA will get Medicaid, and will be underinsured in many states.[26]

• *Profiteering, with the business model trumping service to patients*

The largest five private insurers in the country paid out $12.2 billion in profits to investors in 2009, a year when 2.7 million

Americans lost their health coverage;[27] profits of WellPoint (now renamed as Anthem), the nation's second largest insurer, climbed by 24 percent in the second quarter of 2013 as its stock reached an all-time high;[28] in the last three years, 32 executives of the nation's largest for-profit insurers have received a total of $548.4 million in cash and stock options.[29]

- *Inadequate accountability or regulation of premiums*

Oversight and regulatory effectiveness varies widely from one state to another, and tends to be friendly to insurers. And the insurance industry lobbies hard to keep it that way. In California, for example, the five largest insurers (Anthem/WellPoint, Blue Shield of California, Kaiser Foundation Health Plan, Health Net, and United-Healthcare), spent tens of millions of dollars in opposition to Proposition 45 on the State ballot, which would have given state regulators the ability to reject rate increases deemed excessive.[30] They were successful as this initiative went down to defeat in the midterm elections.

- *Gaming the ACA for profits more than service to patients*

Here we have many examples, starting with Medicare Advantage, with many insurers being cited by CMS for serious violations of Medicare's patient protection requirements, including inappropriate denial of coverage and failure to consider physicians' clinical information.[31] Many plans have gamed risk assessment measures by claiming that patients are sicker than they are, thereby receiving $122.5 billion in overpayments since 2004.[32] In seven major U.S. cities, one-half of bronze plans will require enrollees to pay the deductible (often $5,000) before covering a doctor's visit.[33] Some insurers are selling short-term plans that last less than 12 months, evading any of the ACA's requirements.[34]

• *Non-profit health insurance cooperatives haven't met expectations.*

These co-ops were funded by $2 billion under the ACA with the hope that they could inject competition into the on-line insurance marketplaces. However, after the first open enrollment ended, 14 of the 23 co-ops had enrolled far fewer people than expected, raising questions about their viability and ability to pay back their loans.[35]

5. It is futile to embark on unproven or disproven incremental tweaks to our present system while ignoring health policy and experience around the world.

As the saying goes, it is insanity to keep doing the same things that haven't worked and expect a different result. Yet here we are, laboring on with tweaks of a dysfunctional delivery system and the same flawed multi-payer financing system. Managed care, discredited from our experience in and after the 1990s, is back in privatized Medicaid plans. Cost-sharing by patients is increasing for the newly insured as well as those with existing insurance. Pay-for-performance, although still unproven, is a big part of the ACA's hopes to contain costs and improve quality through accountable care organizations (ACOs). Meanwhile, all the Republicans can offer is to defund parts of the ACA, or repeal it altogether. The Patient Choice, Affordability, Responsibility, and Empowerment (CARE) Act, proposed in early 2014 by three Republican senators, would repeal the ACA, further privatize health care, and include other warmed-over failed ideas such as vouchers and health savings accounts.[36]

Meanwhile, our policy makers and politicians, following the money, keep relying on markets and ignoring the lessons of virtually all industrialized nations around the world that have found fundamental financing reform necessary to assure access to care and containment of health care costs.

In their excellent 2014 book, *Social Insurance: America's Neglected Heritage and Contested Future*, Theodore Marmor,

Ph.D., professor emeritus of public policy and management at Yale University, with his co-authors Jerry Mashaw and John Pakutka, have this to say on the subject:

> *Broadening health insurance coverage to include more than 50 million Americans is a worthy goal—as is any attempt to get a handle on cost inflation in health care expenses in the United States. But we believe that the idea that these goals are best pursued through market-mimicking and means-tested social programs is profoundly misguided. Fragmented risk pools will not promote either perceptions of fairness or us-us politics in the provision of health insurance. And patient choice and competition among insurers has no demonstrated record of cost control in medical care either in the United States or elsewhere in the developed world.*[37]

6. In order to gain the most efficiency of insurance coverage, we need the largest possible risk pool to spread the risk and avoid adverse selection.

By leaving the 1,300 some private insurers responsible for financing much of our health care system, the architects of the ACA swept aside any chance of gaining efficiency of insurance coverage because it made inevitable continued and increased fragmentation of risk pools.

The larger and more diverse the risk pool is, the more efficient insurance can be in having healthier people share the costs of sicker people and keeping insurance affordable. The mathematics of risk pools have been well known for years. According to the National Institute for Health Care Management, 5 percent of the population accounts for nearly one-half of all health care spending; 15 percent of the population used no care in the last year studied. Put another way, we have the *20-80 Rule*, which states that 20 percent of the population is responsible for 80 percent of all health care spending. There are two main implications from these figures, as quoted from the above source:

1. *With half the population incurring just $36 billion in health care costs, it simply is not possible to realize significant contemporaneous or short-term savings by directing cost-control efforts at this group.*
2. *Emerging payment and delivery system reforms, such as accountable care organizations, rely on integrated provider organizations to accept some degree of risk for a defined patient population. These organizations will need a patient base that is large enough to balance out the sizable downside risk of attracting just a few high-spending cases.*[38]

Despite assurances from the ACA's supporters, there is no way that it can develop a big enough risk pool to avoid adverse selection, given the motivations of the private insurance industry and the predictable behavior of markets. That is especially true because younger, healthier people are not signing up in droves on the exchanges, partly for reasons of premium costs for plans of low actuarial value. It's also not just the young who are not signing up—a recent national study by Bankrate found that one-third of men between the ages of 50 and 64 were opting to stay uninsured.[39] The potential risk pool under the ACA will suffer another drop as many Americans request exemptions from the individual mandate. HHS has released a list of at least a dozen reasons that individuals can request exemptions, such as being homeless or having filed for bankruptcy in the last six months. It expects at least 12 million people to file for exemptions.[40]

7. The ACA is a massive bailout of private interests profiting on the backs of sick or injured Americans.

The aforementioned Professor Field gets it right in his new book, *Mother of Invention*, with this accurate overview of the ACA:

> *The ACA set the stage for a financial boon for the health care industry in numerous ways. It enables millions of new customers to purchase individual policies. It permits*

Medicaid programs in many states to retain more managed care companies to administer benefits. It helps hospitals and many physicians to realize increased revenues by giving more of their patients access to the financial resources needed to pay for care. And, over time, countless other businesses will emerge and thrive under the ACA's government-created structure as the ingenuity of the private sector finds ways to thrive off its new public base.[41]

Here are just three of many perks served up by the government to feed this burgeoning health care industry:

- Large insurers such as WellPoint (Anthem) and Humana can expect to gain $5.5 billion in 2015 through the "risk corridor program" to cover "losses"; the ACA fully protects insurers from losses even as it gives them expanded markets.[42]
- New armies of "navigators" are needed to help guide confused millions through the hoops of the exchanges, leading to another increase in insurance premiums.[43]
- Big increases in information technology, including e-health, which will help enrollees find policies, at a six-percent commission for each policy sold.

8. The single-payer alternative was considered "politically unfeasible" by being "too disruptive" to the existing system; instead, look at how disruptive the ACA has been compared to the simplified single-payer alternative.

This is what President Obama said in defense of the ACA in November 2013:

What we did was we chose a path that was least disruptive to try to finally make sure that health care is treated in this country like it is in every other advanced country: That it's not some privilege that just a certain portion of people can have, but it's something that everybody has some confidence about. . . And, you know we didn't go far left and choose an

176

*approach that would have been much more disruptive. We
didn't adopt some more conservative proposals that would
have been much more disruptive.*[44]

Disruptive to whom is the question raised by these state-ments. These words, of course, represent a value judgment as well as lack of historical awareness of how incremental tweaks of the market-based system have failed for so many years. The funda-mental question remains: who is our health care system for? If we answer, "for patients and their families," then we would want to select a way to achieve universal coverage for comprehensive care for all Americans that is most affordable for everyone—with-out the profit motive, perverse incentives, and waste that meet the needs of corporate stakeholders.

The president, his advisors, and influential policy makers, typically with close ties to corporate America, also defend their choices as being more "politically feasible" than single-payer would have been, again ignoring many polls over the years that have shown a majority of Americans favoring a system of univer-sal access to national health insurance. Kip Sullivan, an attorney and health policy expert, brings us these useful insights related to how we might best define political feasibility:

*Any legislation that proposes to achieve universal coverage,
or even to cut the uninsured rate substantially, is not
politically feasible, or at a minimum is no more feasible than
single-payer legislation, if: (1) it doesn't simultaneously
reduce health care spending; or (2) is so complex it cannot
be implemented within a reasonable period of time; and (3)
once the bill is enacted, is it politically sustainable?*[45]

It is hard to imagine a more disruptive situation than we now have with the ACA at its mid-legislative life. We have a very confused and unstable "system," full of discontinuity of in-surance coverage, reduced choices of hospitals and physicians, and uncertainty, with no cost containment in sight. As just one example, most low-income adults who drop below the federal poverty level in states that did not expand Medicaid are finding themselves ineligible for either Medicaid or subsidized coverage on the exchanges.[46] Another example reveals how ineffective accountable care organizations are in containing costs or assuring more coordinated care. A major recent study of 145 organizations participating in Medicare ACO programs found that two-thirds of office visits to specialists were provided *outside* of assigned ACOs, especially for higher-cost patients with more office visits and chronic conditions.[47]

9. The ACA is unaffordable for many patients and their families, is byzantine in its complexity, and is unsustainable in the long run.

We have seen in earlier chapters how prices and costs continue to rise throughout the health care system, how choices about access are being reduced as insurers and hospital systems consolidate, and how complex implementation of the ACA has become. Many employers are dropping coverage, shifting workers to part-time so as to avoid coverage, or transferring them to exchanges. A *Kaiser Health News* analysis found in late 2013 that 18 percent of U.S. counties had only one insurer offering plans, with one-third of counties having only two insurers involved.[48] Eligibility for private and public programs remains in flux, depending on employment, income, age, geographical location, level of state participation in Medicaid, immigration status, and other factors. We have also seen a series of delays, with loosening of the ACA's standards for both the employer and individual mandates.

As many tens of millions of Americans know full well, even if they have had or gain new insurance coverage, they are responsible for rising deductibles, co-payments and out-of-pocket costs. Insurers have been quick to offer limited plans on the exchanges with small networks of physicians and hospitals. Reacting to widespread public backlash reminiscent of that to managed care in the 1990s, the federal government set new standards in October 2013 setting higher standards for the federal exchanges in 36 states that serve two-thirds of the country's population. These standards, still quite loose in requiring insurers to have contracts with at least 30 percent of "essential community providers" in their service area, drew immediate concerns from America's Health Insurance Plans (AHIP). The U.S. Chamber of Commerce labeled these requirements a "regulatory power grab" as it warned of increased costs that would result.[49]

Meanwhile, most of the ACA's $1 trillion in subsidies is going to the insurance industry as an enormous transfer of public wealth to private hands. Since the ACA was enacted, the average stock price of the big for-profit health insurers has doubled, and the top 10 insurers have spent some $25 billion on mergers and acquisitions over the past two years.[50]

10. We cannot trust many states to assure an adequate safety net for the uninsured and underinsured.

Although enrollment in Medicaid has increased substantially as a result of the ACA, there are few safeguards in place that will ensure that patients receive adequate care. Many states hire insurance companies to manage care for Medicaid patients in networks of selected physicians and hospitals. Federal rules require these managed care organizations to provide "adequate access to all services covered," but leave it up to the states to define what this means. There are wide variations in definitions from one state to another in terms of numbers of providers and covered services.[51]

The politics of health care, especially in red states and those that have opted out of Medicaid expansion, give us no confidence that the uninsured and underinsured will receive sufficient essential health care. Ironically, the good intentions of the ACA to provide an improved safety net across the country were sidetracked by the U.S. Supreme Court's 2012 ruling to allow states to opt out of Medicaid expansion. These intentions will be compromised in the opt-out states, mostly under Republican leadership.

Before that ruling, the ACA assumed that everyone with incomes below 138 percent of FPL would be covered by Medicaid. Based on that assumption, the ACA will cut by 25 to 50 percent safety net payments to hospitals and health centers for treating the uninsured and underinsured. Payments to physicians will also be cut to such low levels that many physicians will not accept patients on Medicaid.[51]As a result, we can expect many of the most vulnerable among us to be in difficult circumstances, as also happened in Massachusetts after its very similar health care reform act was passed in 2006. A 2013 report comparing safety net hospitals with non-safety net hospitals found that safety net hospitals continued to play a disproportionately large role in caring for disadvantaged patients after reform, and in so doing their financial resources declined as well.[52]

Any gains in coverage through the exchanges or Medicaid will continue to be vulnerable to churning. A recent study estimates that more than 40 percent of adults likely to enroll in Medicaid or subsidized Marketplace coverage will experience a change in eligibility within 12 months. It further predicts that most adults who lose these subsidies in non-expanding states will become uninsured.[53]

These examples show how draconian the politics have become in some states:

- Republican Governor Nathan Deal of Georgia has refused to expand Medicaid, favors repeal of the ACA, and is even opposed to emergency rooms being open to all comers under the Emergency Treatment and Active Labor Act (EMTALA).[54]
- Despite abortion being a constitutional right of women for the last 41 years, anti-choice groups have forced closure of abortion clinics in many states; in Texas, these closures leave a 400-mile stretch between Houston and the Louisiana border without such a facility.[55]

CONCLUSIONS

From the foregoing, we can see that the Patient Protection and Affordability Care Act (PPACA) is a misnomer. Despite its good intentions about patient protection and affordability of care, it falls far short of universal access, is not restraining the costs of care, and gives the insurance industry many opportunities to game the new system in its own self interest. Costs and prices continue to go up as stakeholders throughout the health care industry profit from new markets. We can anticipate that the cost to patients, families and taxpayers will increase steadily, largely uncontrolled, with no change on the horizon.

Long-term sustainability is therefore a big question. As economist Herbert Stein, Ph.D. has said in what has become known as Stein's Law:

If something cannot go on forever, it will stop.[56]

So let's see in the next chapter what our alternatives are in going forward with health care reform, especially dealing with its financing.

References

1. Scully, T, as cited by Davidson, A. The President wants you to get rich on Obamacare. *The New York Times Magazine*, October 30, 2013.
2. Field, RI. *Mother of Invention: How the Government Created "Free-Market" Health Care*. New York. Oxford University Press, 2014, p. 220.
3. Altman, D. Does the Affordable Care Act cover the uninsured? *Wall Street Journal*, June 19, 2014.
4. Washington Wire. Health insurance. Obamacare states see biggest uninsured drops. *Wall Street Journal*, August 6, 2014.
5. Armour, S. Newly insured face coverage gaps. *Wall Street Journal*, July 8, 2014: A1.
6. Armour, S. Fewer uninsured face fines as health-law waivers swell. *Wall Street Journal*, August 7, 2014.
7. Hamell, L, Rao, M, Levitt, L et al. Survey of non-group health insurance enrollees. *Kaiser Family Foundation*, June 19, 2014.
8. Connor, K. Chief health aide to Baucus is former Wellpoint executive. *Eyes on the Ties* Blog, September 1, 2009.
9. Sirota, D. Thirteen in Congress control health care debate. *Truthout*, August 3, 2009.
10. Center for Public Integrity, as cited by Moyers, B, Winship, M. The unbearable lightness of reform. *Truthout*, March 27, 2010.

11. Fang, L. The shadow lobbying complex, *The Nation*, March10/17, 2014.
12. Suennen, L. Here come the exchanges . . . And the opportunity to turn chaos into gold. *Venture Valkyrie*, October 6, 2013.
13. Soltas, E. Nobody should get rich off Obamacare. *Bloomberg View*, December 3, 2013.
14. Randall, D, Farr, C. In quest for next windfall, tech funds look to healthcare. *Reuters*, September 3, 2014.
15. Plumridge, H, Loftus, P. Inversion frenzy rocks drug sector. *Wall Street Journal*, June 21-22, 2014: B1.
16. Cimilluca, D, Mattioli, D, Walker, J. Taxes fuel medical device merger. *Wall Street Journal*, June 16, 2014: A1.
17. Nichols, L et al. Are market forces strong enough to deliver efficient health care systems? Confidence is waning. *Health Aff (Millwood)* 23 (2): 8-21, 2004.
18. Metz, S. Reducing health care costs: delivery vs. financing approaches. *Health Care Disconnects*, November 12, 2013. (available at www.copernicus-healthcare. org).
19. Radnofsky, L. Health plans to self-renew. *Wall Street Journal*, June 27, 2014: A3.
20. Galewitz, P. Connecticut drops insurers from Medicaid. *Kaiser Health News*, December 29, 2011.
21. Patient advocacy groups. Letter to Sylvia Burwell, Secretary of Health and Human Services, July 28, 2014.
22. Woolhandler, S, Campbell, T, Himmelstein, DU. Costs of health care administration in the United States and Canada. *N Engl J Med* 349: 768-775, 2003.
23. Healthcare-Now! *Single-Payer Activist Guide to the Affordable Care Act*. Philadelphia, PA, 2013, p. 22. Available at www.healthcare-now.org
24. Himmelstein, DU, Thorne, D, Warren, E et al. Medical bankruptcy in the United States, 2007: results of a national study. *Am J Med* 122: 741-746, 2009.
25. Andrews, M. Proposal to add skimpier 'copper' plans to marketplace raises concerns. *Kaiser Health News*, July 1, 2014.
26. Galewitz, P, Fleming, M. 13 states aim to limit Medicaid. *USA Today*, July 24, 2012.
27. Health Care for America Now. Health insurers break profit records as 2.7 million Americans lose coverage. 2010. Available a http://hcfan.3cdn.net/ a9ce29d.3038ef8a1r1_dhm6b9q01.pdf
28. Associated Press. Wellpoint's 2nd quarter profit soars 24 pct; insurer details overhaul growth possibilities. *Washington Post Business*, July 24, 2013.
29. UNITE HERE. The irony of Obamacare, March 2014.
30. Potter, W. Insurers using familiar playbook to protect profits. *The Progressive Populist*, October 1, 2014, p. 10.
31. Pear, R. U.S. finds many failures in Medicare health plans. *New York Times*, October 12, 2014.
32. Outrage of the Month: Medicare Advantage—Whose advantage? *Health Letter*. Public Citizen 29(6), June 2013.
33. Appleby, J. Consumers beware: Not all health plans cover a doctor's visit before the deductible is met. *Kaiser Health News*, December 23, 2013.

34. Andrews, M. Short-term plans can skirt health law requirements. *Kaiser Health News*, October 28, 2013.

35. Radnofsky, L. Mixed bag for health co-ops. *Wall Street Journal*, June 12, 2014: A3.

36. Coburn, T. Dr. Coburn unveils Obamacare replacement - Patient CARE Act - with Senators Burr and Hatch. January 27, 2014. Available at: htpp://www. coburn.senate.gov/public/index.cfm/pressreleases?ContentRecord id=bd2f1e3a-3c25-4ea2-80a0-25b0753bcc6a

37. Marmor, TR, Mashaw, JL, Pakutka, J. *Social Insurance: America's Neglected Heritage and Contested Future.* Los Angeles. Sage Publications Inc., 2014. p. 238.

38. National Institute for Health Care Management. A comparatively small number of sick people account for most health care spending, August 2, 2012.

39. Flavelle, C, Obamacare's dropouts are middle-age men. *Bloomberg News*, March 17, 3014.

40. Jost, T. Implementing health reform: the state of the exchanges, income verification, and more. *Health Affairs blog*, October 16, 2013.

41. Ibid # 2, pp. 220-221.

42. Wayne, A. Insurers' Obamacare losses may reach $5.5 billion in 2015. *Bloomberg News Businessweek*, March 4, 2014.

43. Aizenman, NC. For insurance exchanges, states need "navigators"—and hiring them is a huge task. *Washington Post*, February 4, 2013.

44. Obama, B. As cited by Daily Kos member. Single-payer "disruptive," Mr. President? Only to insurance companies' profits. *Daily Kos*, November 14, 2013.

45. Sullivan, K. Comment on Quote-of-the-Day. Was the ACA "politically feasible?" January 31, 2014.

46. Sommers, BD, Graves, JA, Swartz, K et al. Medicaid and marketplace eligibility changes will occur often in all states; policy options can ease impact. *Health Affairs*, April 2014.

47. McWilliams, JM, Chernew, ME, Dalton, JB et al. Outpatient care patterns and organizational accountability in Medicare. *JAMA Internal Medicine*, April 21, 2014.

48. Rau, J, Appleby, J. Marketplace plans vary widely in costs, within counties and across the country. *Kaiser Health News*, October 4, 2013.

49. Pear, R. White House tightens health plan's standards after consumers complain. *New York Times*, March 14, 2014.

50. UNITE HERE. The irony of Obamacare: making inequality worse. New York, NY. March 7, 2014.

51. Pear, R. For many new Medicaid enrollees, care is hard to find, report says. *New York Times*, September 27, 2014.

52. Mohan, A, Grant, J, Batalden, M, McCormick, D. The health of safety net hospitals following Massachusetts health care reform: changes in volume, revenue, costs, and operating margins from 2006 to 2009. *Int J Health Services* 43 (2): 321-335, 2013.

53. Sommers, BD, Graves, JA, Swartz, K et al. Medicaid and marketplace eligibility changes will occur often in all states; policy options can ease impact. *Health Affairs* 33 (4): 700-707, April 2014.

54. Lewison, J. Here's one Republican plan to reduce health care costs. *Daily Kos,* February 26, 2014.
55. CBS/Associated Press. 400-mile stretch of Texas now without an abortion clinic. March 6, 3014.
56. Stein, H. htpp://en.wikipedia.org/wiki/Herbert_Stein

Part Three

THE SINGLE-PAYER ALTERNATIVE: NATIONAL HEALTH INSURANCE

[We have created] a society in which materialism dominates moral commitment, in which the rapid growth that we have achieved is not sustainable environmentally or socially, in which we do not act together as a community to address our common needs, partly because rugged individualism and market fundamentalism have eroded any sense of community and have led to rampant exploitation of unwary and unprotected individuals and to an increasing social divide. There has been an erosion of trust—and not just in our financial institutions. It is not too late to close these fissures.[1]

—Joseph Stiglitz, Ph.D., Nobel laureate in economics, former chief economist at the World Bank, and author of *Free Fall: America, Free Markets, and the Sinking of the World Economy*

All things are possible until they are proven impossible— and even the impossible may be only so, as of now.[2]

—Pearl S. Buck, first American woman to win the Nobel Prize for Literature, and author of the Pulitzer Prize winning *The Good Earth* and *A Bridge for Passing*

References

1. Stiglitz, JE. *Freefall: America, Free Markets, and the Sinking of the World Economy.* New York. W.W Norton & Company, 2010, pp. 275-276.

2. Buck, PS. *BrainyQuote.*

CHAPTER 11

FINANCIAL REFORM: MULTI-PAYER VS. SINGLE-PAYER

The ACA may be the last bad idea that Americans try;
after it fails, we will finally do the right thing: single-payer
health insurance.[1]

—Gerald Friedman, Ph.D., professor of economics,
University of Massachusetts

As we have seen in foregoing chapters, we cannot expect to reform the delivery system for U.S. health care without changing the way we finance care. So far, we have taken incremental steps that leave multi-payer financing in place, with some 1,300 private insurers as mostly for-profit middlemen between physicians and other providers and patients. Earlier chapters make the case that the ACA, the latest iteration in incremental reform, will not achieve universal access, contain costs or prices, or assure a comprehensive set of benefits for our population.

Therefore, we now have to ask fundamental questions about how to better finance health care. Should we seek a not-for-profit system that assures universal access to all Americans in a single risk pool that is the most efficient, fair and sustainable for the long-term? Or should we perpetuate a failing multi-payer, private financing system that is only still alive through taxpayer subsidy dollars? The answer should by now be obvious, but let's compare these alternatives.

This chapter has three goals: (1) to compare two basic models of health care financing—multi-payer vs. single-payer; and (2) to discuss the extent to which the ACA has been a political hot potato; and (3) to briefly consider whether the ACA can be a bridge to a single-payer system.

MULTI-PAYER AND THE ACA
VS. SINGLE-PAYER FINANCING

Earlier chapters have described how the present multi-payer system under the ACA is functioning. A March 2014 hearing by the U.S. Senate's Committee on Health, Education, Labor and Pensions (HELP) gives us an overview of some major features of single-payer financing from experience around the world. These excerpts from an opening statement by Tsung-Mei Cheng, LL.B, M.A., health policy research analyst at Princeton University's Woodrow Wilson School of Public and International Affairs, shows how different single-payer financing would be compared to what we have now:[2]

1. *If equity and social solidarity in access to health care and financing health care were fundamental goals of a health care system, the single-payer system provides an ideal platform for achieving these goals.*
2. *Single-payer systems typically are financed by general or payroll taxes in a way that tailors the individual's or family's contribution to health care financing to their ability to pay, rather than to their health status.*
3. *These systems protect individual households from financial ruin due to medical bills.*
4. *Single-payer health systems typically afford patients free choice of health care provider . . . Most Americans are confined to networks of providers for their insurance policy. They appear to have traded freedom of choice among providers for the sake of choice among insurers.*
5. *In single-payer systems "money follows the patient." Therefore providers of health care must and do compete for patients on the basis of quality and patient satisfaction, but not price.*
6. *In a single-payer health insurance system, health insurance is fully portable from job to job and into unemployment status and retirement. The "job-lock" problem prevalent in the U.S. is unknown in these systems, contributing to labor-market efficiency.*

7. *Because all funds to providers of health care in a single-payer system flow from one payer, it is relatively easy to control total health spending in such systems. . . . Provider inputs are part of formal negotiations over health care budgets.*

8. *For the most part, single-payer systems achieve their cost control by virtue of the monopsonistic market power they enjoy vis a vis providers of health care.*

The ACA, based as it is on subsidized continuation of multiple private insurers, brings us restricted choices of physicians and hospitals, and in some cases of insurers, as in rural areas. We will fall short of universal access, grow the ranks of the underinsured, and still restrict some essential services based on ability to pay—a cruel form of rationing. While the ACA requires insurers to offer ten categories of essential services (such as primary care, emergency care and hospital care), they are already gaming the new marketplace in ways that restrict coverage. President and CEO of America's Health Insurance Plans (AHIP), Karen Ignagni, is even proposing a fifth tier of coverage (less than bronze), which would *not* have to cover all ten categories of care. Disingenuously, she makes her argument in terms of adding choice to consumers:

> *If you take ten categories of coverage and you have a giant step up, that is a bridge too far for some individuals. . . . So I would create a lower tier so that people could gradually get into the program, so they could be part of the risk pool so we don't hold the healthier people outside, so the process could be working the way it was designed, so we get the healthy and the sick. . . . What I would do is give people more choices. . . . They're in control if they have more choices.*[3]

As a result of this "grand bargain" between the architects of the ACA and the corporate stakeholders in our medical-industrial complex, consumer protection remains elusive. A recent study by the Kaiser Family Foundation finds that one in three Americans still have difficulty paying their medical bills, and that medical debt has these serious consequences: difficulty accessing care, damaged credit, emotional distress, depleted long-term assets, housing instability, economic deprivation, and bankruptcy. The study identifies these ways that medical debt becomes a problem for people *with health insurance*:

- *In network cost-sharing*
- *Medical bills high relative to income and savings*
- *Cost-sharing "multipliers"*
- *Treatments spanning two plan years (doubles cost-sharing)*
- *Family-level cost-sharing (2 family members doubles cost-sharing)*
- *Cost-sharing for chronic conditions (cost-sharing)*
- *Extremely high cost-sharing (deductibles may not apply to out-of-pocket limits)*
- *Out-of-network care*
- *Fewer cost-sharing protections (e.g. no out-of-pocket limits)*
- *"Inadvertent" out-of-network care*
- *Balance billing (paying balances exceeding allowed charges)*
- *Health plan coverage limits or exclusions*
- *Unaffordable premiums*

Looking forward as the ACA becomes fully implemented, the authors draw this conclusion:

In light of the limited assets many people have, the problem of medical debt is likely to persist and lead to continued debate over the tradeoffs inherent in providing more comprehensive coverage and limiting federal costs for premium and cost-sharing subsidies.[4]

As comprehensive coverage falls victim to limited benefit policies and others with restricted benefits marketed by the now-subsidized private insurance industry, Figure 11.1 illustrates a common problem for the underinsured.

FIGURE 11.1

Your Coverage Doesn't Seem to Include Illness

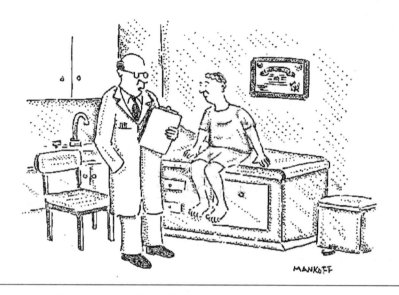

Reprinted with permission from Robert Mankoff.

Gerald Friedman, Ph.D., brings us this important insight into what the ACA is doing:

Subsidized coverage expansion and restrictions on insurance company abuses are significant gains. But these gains come at a steep price because with the ACA the Obama administration has entrenched the insurance and drug companies as arbiters of America's health care system. This is not only repugnant because of these companies' abusive policies, but it endangers everything that the ACA seeks because it precludes effective action to contain rapidly rising health care costs. Private plans divert health care spending into channels that do nothing to actually deliver health care, such as advertising and profit. The proliferation of plans has also raised billing costs for providers, hospitals, clinics, and private medical practices, costs that now come to nearly a third of the cost of health care. Without effective controls on profit and administrative costs, health care costs will continue to soar, rising faster than household, company and government budgets. The pressure to control health care costs will continue and, having removed profits and administrative waste from consideration, the ACA risks becoming a vehicle to control health care costs by squeezing providers and restricting access.[5]

Even with the employer and individual mandates, the ACA remains voluntary to a considerable extent, given the exclusions and delays for each and the relatively light penalties for non-compliance. Because of the adverse selection that is inevitable in the new insurance market, we can expect the cost of premiums to continue to climb, and become less affordable for many individuals and families. As Marmor, Mashaw and Pakutka argue in their recent book, *Social Insurance: America's Neglected Heritage and Contested Future*:

If anyone is to be insured at reasonable cost, it is typically necessary that everyone, or nearly everyone, be compelled to be insured through a publicly mandated program.[6]

In order to keep their premiums lower, insurers have designed narrow networks of physicians and hospitals. A March 2014 report by the Associated Press found that only four of 19 nationally recognized cancer centers said that patients have access to them through all the insurers in their state exchanges. Dan Mendelson, CEO of the market research firm Avalere Health, comments:

This is a marked deterioration of access to the premier cancer centers for people who are signing up for these plans.[7]

Continuing with the example of cancer patients, the prices of cancer drugs in today's system have soared out of sight. Twelve of the 13 new cancer drugs approved in 2012 were priced at more than $100,000 a year. With a 20 percent co-payment, these drugs are unaffordable even for well-insured patients. This problem is even more disturbing when we consider that only one of these 12 drugs provides survival of more than 2 months.[8] With a national health program, we would have two main ways to make these drugs both more affordable and effective—by price reductions through bulk purchasing and an evidence-based process that would assess drugs based on length of survival and quality of life.

Table 11.1 compares and contrasts the differences between the multi-payer ACA and single-payer financing through a national health insurance plan. Figure 11.2 draws the same comparison in terms of complexity vs. simplicity.

TABLE 11.1

THE ACA VS. SINGLE-PAYER NATIONAL HEALTH INSURANCE

ACA	NHI
At least 31 million uninsured in 2024	Universal coverage when enacted
Employment and Medicaid based, with subsidies for many millions	Covers all ages regardless of work status, gender, etc.
Variable coverage and benefits	Comprehensive benefits
Multi-tiered system, based on ability to pay	Single standard for all, based on medical need
Limited choice of doctor and hospital	Free choice of doctor and hospital
Fragmented, inefficient risk pools	One big, efficient risk pool
Large intrusive bureaucracy	Administrative simplicity
For-profit business ethic	Service ethic
No cost containment	Cost containment through negotiated fees, budgets and prices
Unsustainable	Sustainable through progressive taxes; employers and individuals pay less than they do now

FIGURE 11.2

Simplicity, Anyone?

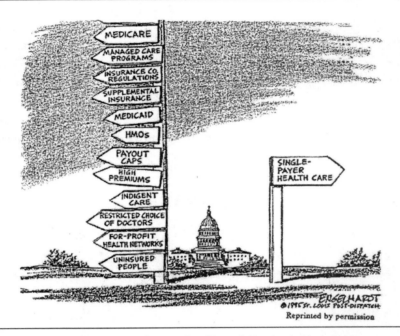

© copyright 1995 Englehardt in the *St. Louis Post Dispatch.* Reprinted with permission

Given increased gaming of the ACA by insurers with minimal regulation by government, we can anticipate continued increases in the numbers of underinsured. That problem would go away immediately with enactment of single-payer national health insurance.

How to pay physicians remains a challenging problem regardless of the financing system. As we have seen earlier, over treatment by physicians and other providers has been a big problem for many years, with up to one-third of health care services either inappropriate or unnecessary. Fee-for-service (FFS) has played a large role in this problem. The managed care "revolution" of the late 1980s and 1990s sought to control this problem through health maintenance organizations (HMOs) and capitation payments to physicians caring for a population of patients. But that strategy was soon discredited as the public revolted against restricted choices and denial of services, realizing that fee-for-*non service* was worse than FFS.

Today's version of the HMO strategy under the ACA brings us accountable care organizations (ACOs), bundled payments, pay-for-performance, and risk assessment metrics, all unproven as ways to contain costs and reduce over-utilization of health care services. Now we are seeing new, ingenious ways to pad the bottom line of revenues for hospitals and physicians, especially through "upcoding" of diagnoses and severity of illness. As Drs. Himmelstein and Woolhandler point out in their excellent recent article, risk-assessment tools and quality metrics are still not up to the job of reining in the profit motive of hospital systems and physicians. In their words:

> *In the profit-maximizing milieu of American medicine, capitation risks make things even worse. "Risk-sharing" too often means that physicians earn bonuses for denying care—a danger perceived by patients, who take a dim view of capitation. Risk-sharing is not simply the inverse of fee-for-service, but of fee-splitting, the illegal practice of kickbacks for referrals.*[9]

By contrast, how would physicians be paid, and how would they fare, under single-payer NHI? Present reimbursement methods, such as those existing under the ACA and the AMA's dominant role through their previously mentioned RUC process, would be abandoned. We could expect that an increasing number of physicians would be salaried in group practices, often as part of hospital systems. The government would negotiate fees with physician organizations, rebalancing differences between primary care, psychiatry and other time-intensive specialties and the more procedure-oriented specialties. We could anticipate higher reimbursement for the former and reduced reimbursement to the latter group, many of whom are already over compensated. The situation of primary care physicians, as the most critical shortage group, would be much improved, with reduced practice overheads and more time for direct patient care. Looking to other countries with single-payer universal coverage systems, such as Canada and the United Kingdom, primary care physicians would receive considerably higher incomes than they do today.

THE ACA AS A POLITICAL HOT POTATO

The ACA, or Obamacare, was a polarizing issue throughout the 2014 midterm campaigns, with bipartisanship nowhere to be seen. Republicans were opposed in principle to the ACA as a government takeover and disruption of markets even as corporate stakeholders were profiting in new ways from expanded markets. There was no recognition that government subsidies were propping up private insurers, that drug companies could continue to charge what the market will bear for their drugs, or that the ACA was actually drafted along long-standing conservative principles. The right was holding fast to long-held views that individuals must be responsible for their own lot, that they should have "skin in the game" as "empowered consumers" shopping on health care markets, and that the role of health insurance should be more protection against catastrophic costs than comprehensive. In so doing, they accepted a system based on ability to pay, not medical need, and that we are not all in the same boat concerning our individual vulnerability to bankrupting medical bills.

Politicians on the right called for repeal of the ACA, using it as a hostage in horse-trading over other issues, or defunding key parts of the bill. As they did so, they had little new to offer of their own as an alternative. They were torn between trying to craft a comprehensive bill or offering up bills dealing with such small-bore measures as allowing purchase of health insurance policies across state lines or expanding access to health savings accounts.[10]

In the 2014 midterm election campaigns took shape, Democrats running for election found themselves in the hot seat. If they abandoned their party's signature domestic achievement of Obama's first term, they would be vulnerable to attacks and demagoguery from the right. Yet they had to be increasingly aware of public polling against the bill, and perhaps were becoming more uncertain as to its future capacity to bring broad access to more affordable health care of higher quality. Some Democrats facing re-election battles considered bringing bills forward to "fix" some of the ACA's problems, such as offering a "copper" plan with lower premiums and higher out-of-pocket costs than the bronze plan.[11]

It is striking how the debate in Congress across party lines has so much in common and still fails to consider major financing reform. The ACA is built on conservative principles from the right, including means-testing, privatizing, and decentralization to the states. As Michael Lind, author of *Land of Promise: An Economic History of the United States* and co-founder of the New America Foundation, warns:

> [If the ACA] *is treated by progressives as the greatest liberal public policy success in the last half-century, then how will progressives be able to argue against proposals by conservative Republicans and center-right neoliberal Democrats to means-test, privatize and decentralize Social Security and Medicare in the years ahead? . . . The real 'suicide caucus' may consist of those on the center-left who, by passionately defending the Affordable Care Act rather than holding their noses, are unwittingly reinforcing the legitimacy of the right's long-term strategy of repealing the greatest achievements of American liberalism.*[12]

History is likely to look back on these years as ones of timidity of most Democrats in failing to take on real financing reform of U.S. health care. If they had been willing to buck the political power and money of corporate stakeholders in perpetuating unfettered markets and rally for single-payer as the better alternative with long-standing majority public support, they could well have been the dominant party for years to come.

CAN THE ACA BE A BRIDGE TO SINGLE-PAYER?

This question has been asked by many. As we see from the above, however, the ACA is fundamentally different from NHI, so that it cannot lead to national health insurance except by how we respond to its failures. Dr. Don McCanne answers the question this way:

The incremental path to single-payer through Obamacare has no bridge across the chasm. It would be a tragedy to spend a decade or two, standing on one edge of the chasm, looking across and trying to figure out how legislative patches can build a bridge to the other side, when patches cannot repair a bridge that doesn't even exist. Only a new infrastructure will do. We must begin building a single-payer system with all due haste.[13]

Dr. Margaret Flowers, pediatrician and health policy expert, clarifies the important question before us:

The most important conversation we should be having right now in the United States is not how many people are insured, knowing that insurance is not protective; it's: do we want to continue to treat healthcare as a commodity where people only get what they can afford, or do we want to join the rest of the industrialized nations in the world and treat healthcare as a public good and create a system where people can get what they need?[14]

What we end up doing remains a political question. As Dr. Marcia Angell, senior lecturer in social medicine at Harvard Medical School and former editor of the *New England Journal of Medicine*, observes:

My fervent hope is that as the ACA unravels and costs go up, the U.S. will finally be ready to embrace a nonprofit single-payer system that covers everyone, from the president on down. My fear, however, is that Americans will instead conclude that providing universal health care is simply too expensive, and give up on it. The tragedy in that case would be that the country was too insular and too much in the pocket of the health industry to recognize that universal care can be provided relatively cheaply, as other countries have shown.[15]

References

1. Friedman, G. The last bad idea: The Patient Protection and Affordable Care Act. The Center for Popular Economics: Economics for People, not Profits, August 23, 2013.
2. United States Senate. Committee on Health, Education, Labor and Pensions (HELP), Subcommittee Hearing— Access and Cost: What the U.S. Health Care System Can Learn from Other Countries. March 11, 2014.
3. Ignagni, K. Newsmakers. C-SPAN, March 21,2014.
4. Pollitz, K, Cox, C, Lucia K et al. Medical debt among people with health insurance. *Kaiser Family Foundation,* January 2014.
5. Ibid # 1.
6. Marmor, TR, Mashaw, JL, Pakutka, J. *Social Insurance: America's Neglected Heritage and Contested Future*, Los Angeles. Sage Publications, 2014, p. 218.
7. Alonzo-Zaldivar, R. Health law concerns for cancer centers. *Associated Press,* March 19, 2014.
8. Light, DW, Kantarjian, H. Market spiral pricing of cancer drugs. *Cancer,* November 15, 2013.
9. Himmelstein, DU, Woolhandler, S. Global amnesia: embracing fee-for-non-service—again. *J Gen Internal Med,* January 7, 2014.
10. Newhauser, D. GOP leaders huddle on Obamacare alternative. *Roll Call,* February 25, 2014.
11. Peterson, K. Democrats weigh health-law fixes. *Wall Street Journal,* March 27, 2014.
12. Lind, M. Here's how GOP Obamacare hypocrisy backfires. *Salon,* October 28, 2013.
13. McCanne, D. Quote-of-the-Day, October 21, 2013.
14. Flowers, M. As quoted in Climate Catastrophe Now + The Most Important Question about Obamacare. *Nation of Change,* April 20, 2014.
15. Angell, M. Patients and profits. Presentation at the annual meeting of Physicians for a National Health Program, Boston, MA, November 2, 2013.

CHAPTER 12

THREE COMPELLING ARGUMENTS
FOR SINGLE-PAYER

*The good old days, when nobody really paid a lot of attention
are gone. We're now front and center in the public policy
sphere . . . What our future holds depends in many ways
on our ability to continue to control the rate of increase of
health care costs . . . It will be a real test over the next five
to eight years as to whether the private sector indeed can
produce the kind of results that would make health care
more affordable.*[1]

—Bernard Tresnowski, president of
Blue Cross Blue Shield, 1994

These words were conveyed in the president's letter to Blue
Cross Blue Shield Association CEOs in 1994, challenging them
and the private sector to make health care more affordable and
casting doubt on their future if that could not be accomplished.
Twenty years have passed, and the outcome of their unsuccessful
collective attempts at cost containment are obvious to us all, even
with the ACA at its legislative mid-life. Less talked about, and
largely proceeding unchallenged, is the premise that health care
is just another commodity for sale on a market where the profit
motive trumps service.

We saw in the last chapter the fundamental differences between multi-payer and single-payer financing of health care, together with the advantages of not-for-profit national health insurance (NHI). But just clarifying these advantages does not carry
the day in overcoming the political power and money that per-
petuates what we have now.

So we need to dig a bit deeper and sort out broad compelling arguments for single-payer financing reform. This chapter will do so in three areas—economic, social-political, and moral.

ECONOMIC ARGUMENT FOR
NATIONAL HEALTH INSURANCE (NHI)

NHI will save money and contain health care costs

We have seen many fiscal studies over the last 20-plus years, both nationally and in many states, that have shown how a system of universal coverage under a single-payer system would save money and contain health care costs. In 1991, the Government Accounting Office (GAO) stated:

If the U.S. were to shift to a system of universal coverage and a single-payer, as in Canada, the savings in administrative costs (10 percent of health spending) would be more than enough to offset the expense of universal coverage.[2]

In 1998, the Economic Policy Institute found that universal coverage could be financed with a 7 percent payroll tax, a 2 percent income tax, and current federal payments for Medicare, Medicaid, and other state and federal government insurance programs. It also acknowledged that:

The impediment to fundamental reform in health care financing is not economic, but political. Political will, not economic expertise, is what will bring about this important change.[3]

In 2005, the National Coalition on Health Care analyzed four different scenarios of health care reform: (1) employer mandates (supplemented with individual mandates if necessary); (2) expansion of existing public programs that cover subsets of the uninsured; (3) creation of new programs targeted at subsets of the uninsured (Federal Employees Health Benefits model); and

(4) establishment of a universal publicly financed program (single-payer). Their report concluded that single-payer would cover comprehensive benefits for all Americans and still save more than $1.1 trillion over the next ten years.[4]

Studies in many states over the last 20 years tell much the same story—insure everyone and still save many millions of dollars. These states include California, Colorado, Delaware, Georgia, Kansas, Maine, Maryland, Massachusetts, Minnesota, Missouri, New Mexico, New York, Rhode Island, and Vermont.[5]

Fast forward to 2013, and we have the classic study of Gerald Friedman, professor of economics at the University of Massachusetts. His extensive study and report concludes that funding *HR 676: The Expanded and Improved Medicare for All Act*, would save an estimated $592 billion annually by cutting the administrative waste of the private health insurance industry ($476 billion) and reducing pharmaceutical prices to European levels ($116 billion). In 2014, the savings would be enough to cover all 44 million uninsured and upgrade benefits for all other Americans, including dental and long-term care. Co-payments and deductibles would be eliminated. Savings would also fund $51 billion in transition costs such as retraining displaced workers and phasing out investor-owned for-profit delivery systems over a 15-year period.

Regressive and obsolete funding sources that total more than $1.72 trillion in 2014 would be replaced by progressive taxation, including a new tax on financial transactions of 0.5 percent per transaction (a so-called Tobin tax), a progressive payroll tax and tax on unearned income, and surtax on high income individuals. (Table 12.1)[6] Although Wall Street interests will lobby against any tax on financial transactions, the U.S. had just such a tax from 1914 to 1966, and 40 countries today have this tax, including the seven with the fastest-growing stock exchanges in the world.[7]

What would this new financing system mean for most of us? The payroll tax would be the main tax for all of us with annual incomes below $225,000—3 percent for those with incomes below $53,000 and 6 percent for those earning more than that. That converts to these kinds of numbers—for annual income of $60,000, $3,600 tax; for $100,000, $6,000 tax; and for $200,000, $12,000 tax. Only five percent of Americans would pay more for insurance under this proposal, which would result in savings for all those with annual incomes up to well above $200,000. (Figure 12.1)

TABLE 12.1

A Progressive Financing Plan For H.R. 676

This plan replaces regressive funding sources and improves and expands comprehensive benefits to all (in billions of dollars).

New progressive revenue sources

• Tobin tax of 0.5% on stock trades and 0.01% per year to maturity on transactions in bond, swaps, and trades.	442
• 6% surtax on household incomes over $225,000	279
• 6% tax on property income from capital gains, dividends, interest, or profits	310
• 6% payroll tax on top 60% with incomes over $53,000	346
• 3% payroll tax on bottom 40% with incomes under $53.000	27
Total new progressive sources	1,404
• Tax expenditure savings	260
• Federal Medicare, Medical, and other health spending, and 20% of current out-of-pocket spending (maintained from current system)	1.454
• Total Revenues	3,113
• Savings for deficit reduction	154

Source: Friedman, G. Funding H.R. 676 The Expanded and Improved Medicare For All Act. How We Can Afford a National Single Payer Health Plan. *Physicians for a National Health Plan*. Chicago, IL, July 31, 2013. Available at htpp://OHR%2067 6_Friedman_7.3.1.13.pdf

Public funding for U.S. health care already covers about 60 percent of total health care costs, if we include taxpayer-paid premiums for private coverage for federal, state, and local government employees. It is more than what other developed countries spend from both public and private sources.[8] These costs would be reduced, leaving a net surplus for deficit reduction of $154 billion in the first year.[9]

FIGURE 12.1

Change in After-Tax Household Income With Single-Payer Health Care

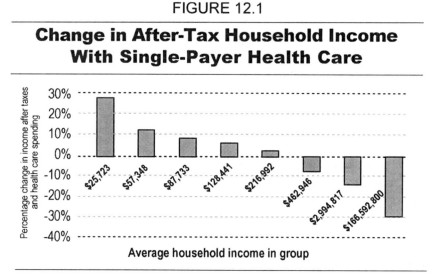

Source: Friedman, G. Funding H.R. 676 *The Expanded and Improved Medicare for All Act. How We Can Afford a National SinglePayer Health Plan.* Physicians for a National Health Plan. Chicago, IL, July 31, 2013. Available at htpp:// 2 OHR%2067 6_Friedman_7.3.1.13.pdf

If Friedman's proposal seems like pie in the sky, other studies in recent years have shown equally persuasive results. A 2012 study, for example, compared health care spending in the U.S. with Canada, which has a single-payer financing system, coupled with a private delivery system, with no co-payments or deductibles. It found that per capita Medicare spending on the elderly since 1980 grew almost three times faster in the United States than in Canada. Medicare would have saved $2 trillion since 1980 if its costs had increased at the same rate as those for seniors in Canada.[10]

The ACA brings out in clear relief what we should have learned many years ago, that the three major dimensions of a health care system—access, cost and quality—are closely interrelated and you can't change one without impacting the others. Just like pinching a balloon—push on one part and it pooches out elsewhere. In this case, the ACA has expanded access through some limited reforms of the private insurance industry and expansion of Medicaid, but prices and costs trend upward without effective cost controls.[11] Meanwhile, quality suffers as insurers push narrowed networks that cause discontinuity and fragmentation of relationships between physicians and patients.

Not only can we expect to pay less for more coverage under single-payer NHI, but we can also expect better quality and outcomes of care with our entire population covered for essential health care. Comprehensive literature reviews in 2002 and 2004 found that for-profit hospitals cost 19 percent more and had 1 to 2 percent higher death rates compared to not-for-profit hospitals.[12,13] We also know that investor-ownership costs more and compromises the quality of care, whether for hospitals, HMOs, dialysis centers, nursing homes, or mental health centers.[14] Investor-owned for-profit health plans, compared to their not-for-profit counterparts, have also been found to have worse quality of care as measured by preventive care, treatment of chronic conditions, and members' access to care.[15] On the opposite end of the spectrum, Veterans Administration hospitals— government-owned and administered with salaried physicians— led the way in implementing electronic medical records. Until the recent scandal involving poor leadership and underfunding, the V.A. had a long record of providing better quality of care with higher patient satisfaction compared to the private sector across the country.[16,17] (Table 12.2)

Other major ways that single-payer NHI can save money compared to our present market-based system are reduction of bureaucracy and waste. Three examples make the point:

- A recent study comparing hospital administrative costs in eight countries found that the U.S. has by far the highest costs—25.3 percent of total hospital expenditures—far higher than any other country. Scotland and Canada, where single-payer systems pay hospitals global operating budgets with separate grants for capital, had the lowest costs, more on the order of about 12 percent.[18] Dr. David Himmelstein, lead author of the study, summed up the differences this way:

  We're squandering $150 billion each year on hospital bureaucracy, and $300 billion more is wasted each year on insurance companies' overhead and the paperwork they inflict on doctors.[19]

TABLE 12.2

Quality of Care in VA Versus Non-VA Hospitals

Health Indicator	VA Score*	National Sample**
Overall	57%	51%
Chronic care	72%	59%
Lung disease	69%	59%
Heart disease	73%	70%
Depression	80%	52%
Diabetes	70%	47%
Hypertension	78%	65%
High cholesterol	64%	53%
Osteoarthritis	65%	57%
Preventive care	64%	44%
Acute care	53%	55%
Screening	68%	46%
Diagnosis	73%	61%
Treatment	56%	41%
Follow-up	73%	58%

Data: RandCorp., Agency for Healthcare Research & Quality

Source: Arnst. C. The best medical care in the U.S. *Business Week*, June 17, 2006

- The Internal Revenue Service has just released forms to be used by employers, insurers, and exchanges for reporting Affordable Care Act tax information to individuals and to the IRS for 2014 and 2015. Some of these forms will be used to determine whether employees have received an affordable and adequate offer of coverage, rendering them ineligible for premium tax credits. Two forms for large employers fill 13 pages with dense, two column print that deal with options for complying with the employer mandate and transition exceptions allowed by the Obama administration.[20] Tax credits vary, of course, with any changes in projected income. It is estimated that one-third of the 7 million households that have received tax credits will be liable for repayments.[21]

- An increasing number of private insurers are now using single-use "virtual credit cards" for claims payments to physicians. In order to process these cards, physicians' office staffs have to plow through detailed instructions, and physicians are then charged additional fees amounting to 3 to 5 percent of their due payments.[22]

One would think that conservatives, based on their professed dedication to efficiency and minimizing bureaucracy, would support the administrative simplicity of single-payer with reduction of waste, instead of typically railing against the alleged burden of government.

As physicians and hospitals transition to a not-for-profit system, the profit motive disappears from the equation, enabling physicians to practice evidence-based medicine free from perverse business incentives and with much less administrative hassle than dealing with our dysfunctional and fragmented multi-payer system. They will even get paid sooner and more predictably without having to pay private insurers part of their reimbursement through virtual credit cards!

Business will do well with NHI, relieved from the burden of providing employer-sponsored health insurance, paying less than it does now, and gaining a healthier workforce. Employers can pocket the present cost of their share of insurance premiums, hire employees based on their qualifications without regard for their health status, and become more competitive in global markets. According to Friedman's analysis, employers would save $31.7 billion in their costs to manage their employer sponsored insurance (ESI) in the first year under NHI, which would shift their payments to payroll taxes—6 percent on the top 60 percent of income earners over $53,000 and 3 percent on the bottom 40 percent earning less than $53,000.

A recent report from Public Citizen, *Severing the Tie That Binds*, identifies three ways that NHI will benefit business: (1) by elimination of "job lock"; (2) by reining in health care costs; and (3) by reducing what businesses pay for health care through a progressive system of taxation that spreads costs more fairly. Taylor Lincoln, research director of Public Citizen's Congress Watch division, states:

Small businesses have rated the cost of health insurance as their top concern for a quarter century, and large businesses struggle with health care obligations that their international competitors do not have to worry about. If it weren't for entrenched partisan alliances, business leaders would have demanded that Congress relieved them of health care burdens long ago.[23]

Since employees typically lose portions of their wages under the present system when employers pay more for their ESI, wages could go up under NHI, thereby permitting many millions of people to better afford goods and services in the overall economy.

Critics of national health insurance raised three questions early on: what would it cost, can we afford it, and what happens to our taxes? Friedman's projections answer all three questions in ways that show that we can get more by paying less by shifting to a universal, not-for-profit system. There is already more than enough money in health care to pay for it—it is just going to the wrong places—profits, inefficiency, and administrative waste. Opposition from the right will argue that U.S. taxes are already too high, and that they must be lowered if we are to stimulate the economy, the old "trickle down" theory. They ignore the fact that top tax rates are now in the 30 percent range compared to more than 60 percent during the Eisenhower years in the 1950s. They also conveniently ignore the fact that personal tax rates in the U.S. today on $100,000 income are hardly that high—55th out of 114 countries around the world.[24]

Under NHI, all Americans will have first dollar coverage without cost-sharing and with full access to physicians and hospitals of their choice. That would be a great leap of progress compared to costs and prices today under the ACA. These are well illustrated by one newly insured patient under Medicaid who went to the doctor for the first time in five years. The charges for his initial visit ($135), his laboratory work ($1,000), and one medication

($300 per month) came to $4,750 over a year. Earning about $10 an hour in his full-time job, he calculated how he would pay that. Working full-time, he earns about $1,600 a month, so it would take him three months to pay the $4,750 bill, which of course does not include the costs of food, housing, transportation and other necessities. Fortunately, he lives in a state that expanded Medicaid, and was newly covered, but in 24 other states, he would have been in dire financial straits.[25] With NHI, the drug's cost would be about 40 percent less through negotiated bulk purchasing by the government.

SOCIAL/POLITICAL ARGUMENT FOR NHI

Growing income inequality among Americans has reached extreme proportions that have put essential health care beyond the reach of the uninsured and the growing ranks of the underinsured. As we have seen, the ACA has improved the situation for some, but the problem grows worse. The numbers are stark, and reminiscent of the Gilded Age more than a century ago. Paul Buchheit, editor and principal author of *American Wars: Illusions and Realities*, recently reported that the richest 400 took in a total of $300 billion in 2013 (an average gain of $750 million for each member of the Forbes 400), a figure larger than the nation's *entire* safety net budget in that year. That 400 own more than $2 trillion among them, more than the holdings of three-fifths of America, or 72 million families.[26] In 2012, the top 10 percent of earners took in more than one-half of the country's total income, the highest level yet recorded. Figure 12.2 shows the share of total income in the U.S. going to the top 1 and 10 percent from 1920 to 2012.[27]

This enormous income gap has serious consequences for most Americans below those stratospheric levels. Figure 12.3, for example, shows how death rates are correlated by income and U.S. zip codes.[28]

Robert Reich, professor of public policy at the University of California Berkeley and chairman of Common Cause, has this to say about where American families find themselves today:

FIGURE 12.2

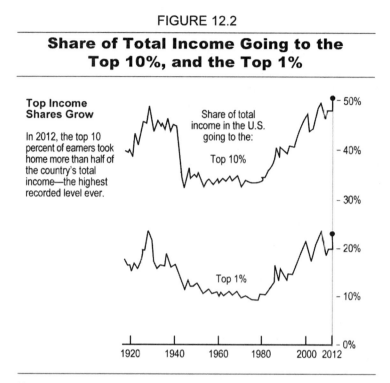

Share of Total Income Going to the Top 10%, and the Top 1%

Top Income Shares Grow

In 2012, the top 10 percent of earners took home more than half of the country's total income—the highest recorded level ever.

Share of total income in the U.S. going to the:

Top 10%

Top 1%

Note: Income is defined as market income and includes capital gains.

Source: Lowrey, A. The rich get richer through the recovery. *New York Times,* September 10, 2013

FIGURE 12.3

Death Rates vs. Income Levels

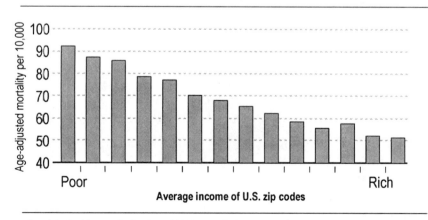

Age-adjusted mortality per 10,000

Poor

Rich

Average income of U.S. zip codes

Reprinted with permission from Wilkinson, R, Pickett, K. *The Spirit Level: Why Greater Equality Makes Societies Stronger.* New York. Bloomsbury Press, 2010, p. 13.

Most American families are worse off today than they were three decades ago. The Great Recession of 2008-2009 destroyed the value of their homes, undermined their savings, and too often left them without jobs. But even before the Great Recession began, most Americans had gained little from the economic expansion that began almost three decades before. Today, the Great Recession notwithstanding, the U.S. economy is far larger than it was in 1980. But where has all the wealth gone? Mostly to the very top.[29]

NHI, or improved and expanded Medicare for All, will eliminate today's multi-tiered health plans that enable insurers to profit from sales of restrictive policies. It will also remove class, gender, and racial disparities in access to care.

If we ask, as we should, whom should the health care system be for, our answer should be—for patients, of course, not for those who profit from our getting sick. In that context, the fairest possible system will be based on medical need, not ability to pay. NHI provides that in a one-tier system. Such a system can also provide the "social glue" that is so important in society, as other advanced nations with universal coverage have found. As Richard Wilkinson and Kate Pickett observe in their excellent book, *The Spirit Level: Why Greater Equality Makes Societies Stronger*:

Changes in inequality and trust go together over the years. With greater inequality, people are less caring of one another, there is less mutuality in relationships, people have to fend for themselves and get what they can—so, inevitably, there is less trust. As de Tocqueville pointed out, we are less likely to empathize with those not seen as equals; material differences serve to divide us socially.[30]

There are, of course, political implications for all of these changes. As Marmor, Mashaw and Pakutka, mentioned in the last chapter, observe:

Social insurance programs engage most of the electorate precisely because they cover common risks and insure most of the population. And because practically everyone is both a contributor and a potential beneficiary, the politics of social insurance tends to be of the "us-us" rather than the "us-them" form. Each individual's sense of earned entitlement or deservingness makes reneging on promises in social insurance programs politically costly. Each individual's responsibility to contribute to the common pool makes extravagant promises of "something-for-nothing" future benefits less politically attractive.[31]

As a result of the widening income gap between the very rich and the rest of us, we now have a plutocracy, as a spate of books have described in recent years. The mainstream media are owned and controlled by corporate money favoring continuation of the status quo. Pushed forward by the *Citizens United* and *McCutcheon* rulings of the U.S. Supreme Court, billionaires and corporate interests are now enabled to buy elections—oligarchy is here. John Nichols and Robert McChesney, authors of their well-documented 2013 book, *Dollarocracy: How the Money and Media Election Complex is Destroying America*, describe the threat to our democracy this way:

The United States has experienced fundamental changes that are dramatically detrimental to democracy. . . . because powerful interests—freed to, in effect, buy elections, unhindered by downsized and diffused media that must rely on revenue from campaign ads—now set the rules of engagement. Those interests so dominate politics that the squabbling of Democrats and Republicans, liberals and conservatives, is a sideshow to the great theatre of plutocracy and plunder. This is not democracy. This is dollarocracy.[32]

Robert Kuttner, co-founder and current co-editor of *The American Prospect* and author of *Everything for Sale: The Virtues and Limits of Markets*, adds this insight:

> *Concentrated wealth translates into concentrated political power. The remedies that could reverse the increasing inequality are outside mainstream politics today, because the wealthy get to define what's mainstream.*[33]

Corporate interests chase profits for their CEOs and share-holders with scant regard for the public they "serve." They exploit loopholes in our tax system as their lobbyists fight against closure of these loopholes. A 2014 report by Citizens for Tax Justice found that over the five-year period 2008-2012, most of our biggest companies weren't paying anywhere near 35 percent of their profits in taxes; 26 companies, including Boeing, General Electric, Priceline.com and Verizon paid no income tax over those five years, despite combined pre-tax profits of $170 billion. Most of the multi-nationals pay lower tax rates here in the U.S. than they pay on their overseas operations.[34] Meanwhile, health care stocks have been outperforming every other sector in the S & P 500, gaining 55 percent in the last two years.[35] Much as we hear from conservatives that those wanting and needing benefits from social programs are "takers", this term can well be applied to corporate America.

If corporate power can be overcome by asserting individual votes over corporate money, changing demographic trends will hopefully improve the odds that NHI be moved to center stage in the political debate as *the* serious alternative to what we now have. Growing minority populations across the country, if their votes can be turned out, can greatly increase the chances for election of liberal and progressive legislators who can enact NHI. And those currently disillusioned citizens of all persuasions also need to vote. That is especially true if we consider that Republicans have no alternative to health care reform except so many already discredited policies of the last 30 years. Figure 12.4 illustrates the gap between the ACA and the Republican "plan."

Given the many problems with the ACA's rollout, delayed signups and problems with the exchanges, and polarized confusion over what the law will and will not do, the electorate was widely split over Obamacare in the 2014 midterms. As one ex-

FIGURE 12.4

Matt Wuerker on Obamacare

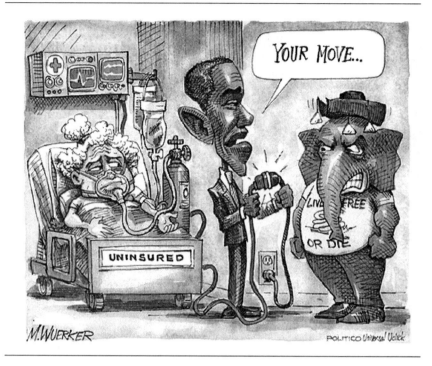

Reprinted with permission from Matt Wuerker

ample, there was a sharp rural-urban division between the parties. Three out of four rural legislators in Congress are Republicans, while urban legislators are evenly represented.[36] Republican candidates were united against the ACA, while Democratic candidates were ambivalent on how much to defend it. Most Democrats couldn't even find the spine to defend the ACA's gradual cuts in overpayments to Medicare Advantage, fearing the wrath of seniors.[37] As Politico reported seven months before the November elections:

Obamacare will be a huge voting issue for Republicans—that's already clear. They'll turn out in droves because they hate the law. What's less clear is how Democrats will get their supporters to the polls to say, "hey, thanks for health reform."[38]

THE MORAL ARGUMENT FOR SINGLE-PAYER

The dominant culture of our market-based health care system treats health care services as commodities, just products in an open market—all about money in a multi-tiered system based on ability to pay. When any of us gets sick or has a major accident, we are brought up short in realizing how unfair, inhumane and cruel the system can be.

These two quotes shine a bright light on the differences between what we have and what other nations have had for many years:

The United States subscribes to a business model that characterizes insurers as commercial entities. Like all businesses, their goal is to make money . . . Under the business model, casual inhumanity is built in and the common good ignored. Excluding the poor, the aged, the disabled, and the ill is sound policy since it maximizes profit. Under the social model, denying coverage to any member of society would refute the fundamental purpose of health insurance.[39]

—Bernard Lown, M.D., professor emeritus at the
Harvard School of Public Health, developer of the cardiac
defibrillator, and co-recipient of the Nobel Peace Prize in
1985 on behalf of International Physicians for
the Prevention of Nuclear War

The most serious problem with [investor-owned] care is that it embodies a new value system that severs the communal roots and Samaritan traditions of hospitals, makes doctors and nurses the instruments of investors and views patients as commodities. In for-profit settings avarice competes with beneficence for the soul of medicine; investor ownership marks the triumph of greed. In our society some aspects of life are off-limits to commerce. We prohibit the selling of children and the buying of wives, juries, and kidneys. Tainted blood is an inevitable consequence of paying blood donors; even sophisticated laboratory tests cannot compensate for blood that is sold rather than given as a gift. Like blood, health care is too precious, intimate, and corruptible to entrust to the market.[40]

—Steffie Woolhandler, M.D. and David Himmelstein, M.D.,
both professors of public health at the City University of
New York and visiting professors of medicine at Harvard
Medical School

When one among us has a major accident or falls prey to a serious illness threatening life and/or bankruptcy, a common and humane response within communities is to launch a collective effort through bake sales or other means to raise money to help a friend or neighbor. These efforts, though laudable, usually fall short of the need and bypass the need for reforming the system itself. Enter the latest response to this need—"crowdfunding", defined by Wikipedia as "the collective effort of individuals who network and pool their money, usually via the Internet, to support efforts initiated by other people or organizations." This has become a new profitable industry of its own as medical fundraising sites on the Internet grow in number and profitability. They charge fees between 3 and 12 percent of the money donated. *GiveForward*, as an example, has raised more than $47 million for families since it began in 2008.[41]

This is not the way it is in almost all advanced countries around the world, where health care is accepted as a human right, not a privilege for those who can pay. The right to health care is still controversial in the U.S., especially among conservatives, and we remain an outlier in the developed world.

As Audrey Chapman, Ph.D., director of the Right to Health Care Project of the American Association for the Advancement of Science (AAAS) said more than 20 years ago:

The right to health care is fundamentally an ethical issue that raises major questions about the relationship and sense of obligation of members of society to each other, and the role of the government in terms of the expectations of the social covenant.[42]

Larry Churchill, Ph.D., professor of medical ethics at Vanderbilt University, brings us these useful qualifying insights:

> *. . . A right to health care based on need means a right to equitable access based on need alone to all effective care society can reasonably afford. . . . Effective care means there is no obligation to provide useless or marginally useful treatments. . . . A right to health care is not a license to demand care. It is not a right to the very best available or even to all one may need. Some very pressing health needs may have to be neglected because meeting them would be unreasonable in the light of other health needs or social priorities.*[43]

Most conservatives in this country oppose the concept of health care as a human right. But this view is not held by conservatives in many other countries around the world. Donald Light, Ph.D. a fellow at the University of Pennsylvania's Center for Bioethics, professor of comparative health care at the University of Medicine and Dentistry of New Jersey, and co-author of the 1996 book, *Benchmarks for Fairness for Health Care Reform*, has found that conservatives and business interests in every other industrialized country have supported universal access to necessary health care on the basis of four conservative moral principles—anti-free-riding, personal integrity, equal opportunity, and just sharing.

He suggests these guidelines for conservatives to stay true to these principles:

1. *Everyone is covered, and everyone contributes in proportion to his or her income.*
2. *Decisions about all matters are open and publicly debated. Accountability for costs, quality and value of providers, suppliers, and administrators is public.*

3. *Contributions do not discriminate by type of illness or ability to pay.*
4. *Coverage does not discriminate by type of illness or ability to pay.*
5. *Coverage responds first to medical need and suffering.*
6. *Nonfinancial barriers by class, language, education, and geography are to be minimized.*
7. *Providers are paid fairly and equitably, taking into account their local circumstances.*
8. *Clinical waste is minimized through public health, self-care, prevention, strong primary care, and identification of unnecessary procedures.*
9. *Financial waste is minimized through simplified administrative arrangements and strong bargaining for good value.*
10. *Choice is maximized in a common playing field where 90-95 percent of payments go toward necessary and efficient health services and only 5-10 percent to administration.*[44]

It is remarkable and surprising that these principles have not yet gained consensus within the business and corporate class as health care becomes ever more expensive, inefficient, unfair and wasteful.

Persuasive as these arguments are for single-payer NHI, we have an ongoing societal blind spot in recognizing and dealing with them. Part of the problem, of course, is the power of corporate and moneyed interests that benefit from the present system. Another part is the myths about single-payer that are promulgated by the opposition, as we will consider in the next chapter.

References

1. Tresnowski, B. President's letter to BCBSA Plan CEOs. June 30, 1994, as cited in: Cunningham, R, III & Cunningham, RJ, Jr. *The Blues: A History of the Blue Cross and Blue Shield System,* DeKalb, IL: Northern Illinois University Press, 1997, pp. 250-251.
2. Canadian Health Insurance: Lessons for the United States. Available at http://archive.gao.gov/d2019/144039.pdf
3. Rasell, E. Universal coverage: how do we pay for it? Available at http://www.epi.org/files/page/-/old/technicalpapers/tp234_1998.pdf
4. Thorpe, KE. National Coalition on Health Care. Impact of Health Care Reform: Projections of costs and savings. 2005. Available at: http://www.latinosnhi.org/pdf/NatCoalitionHC.pdf
5. Hellander, I. Single-payer system cost? Physicians for a National Health Program. Chicago, IL, 2013.
6. Friedman, G. Funding H.R. 676: The Expanded and Improved Medicare for All Act. How We Can Afford a National Single-Payer Health Plan. Physicians for a National Health Plan. Chicago, IL, July 31, 2013. Available at: htpp://www.pnhp.org/sites/default/files/Funding%20HR%20676_Friedman_final_7.31.13.pdf
7. Hightower, J. Tax the churners. *The Progressive,* May 2014, p. 46.
8. Woolhandler, S, Himmelstein, DU. Paying for national health insurance: And not getting it. *Health Aff (Millwood)* 21: 88-98, 2002.
9. Ibid # 6.
10. Himmelstein, DU.Woolhandler, S. Cost control in a parallel universe: Medicare spending in the U.S. and Canada. *Arch Intern Med* online, October 29, 2012.
11. Carroll, AE. Why improving access to health care does not save money. *New York Times,* July 14, 2014.
12. Devereaux, PJ, Heels-Ansdell, D, Lacchetti, C et al. Payments for care at private for-profit and private not-for-profit hospitals: A systematic review and meta-analysis. *CMAJ* 170: 1817-1824, 2004.
13. Devereaux, PJ, Choi, PT, Lachetti, C et al. *CMAJ* 166: 1399-1406, 2002.
14. Geyman, JP. *The Corrosion of Medicine: Can the Profession Reclaim Its Moral Legacy?* Monroe, ME. Common Courage Press, 2008, p. 37.
15. McCue, MJ, Bailit, MH. Assessing the financial health of Medicaid managed care plans and the quality of patient care they provide. New York. The Commonwealth Fund, June 15, 2011.
16. Gaul, GM. Back in the pink: The VA health care system outperforms Medicare and most private plans. *Washington Post National Weekly Edition,* August 29-September 4, 2005, p. 19.
17. Arnst, C. The best medical care in the U.S.: How Veterans Affairs transformed itself—and what it means for the rest of us. *Business Week,* July 17, 2006.

18. Himmelstein, DU, Mun, M, Busse, R et al, A comparison of hospital administrative costs in eight nations: U.S. costs exceed all others by far. *Health Affairs*, September 2014.

19. PNHP press release. Bureaucracy consumes one-quarter of U.S. hospitals' budgets, twice as much as in other nations. Physicians for a National Health Program. Chicago, September 8, 2014.

20. Jost, T. Implementing health reform: Tax Form instructions. *Health Affairs Blog*, August 29, 2014.

21. Alonzo-Zaldivar, R. Tax refunds may get hit due to health law credits. Associated Press, August 24, 2014.

22. AMA Wire. Footing bill for insurers' pay methods shouldn't fall on doctors. Chicago. American Medical Association.

23. Lincoln, T. *Severing the Tie That Binds,* Public Citizen, Washington, D.C., April 2014.

24. Thompson, D. How low are U.S. taxes compared to other countries? *The Atlantic,* January 14, 2013.

25. Daily Kos member. First doctor visit in five years: why Repubs want us broke or dead. *Daily Kos,* March 26, 2014.

26. Buchheit, P. Another shocking wealth grab by the rich, in just one year. *Nation of Change,* January 20, 2014.

27. Lowrey, A. The rich get richer through the recovery. *New York Times,* September 10, 2013.

28. Wilkinson, R, Pickett, K. *The Spirit Level: Why Greater Equality Makes Societies Stronger.* New York. Bloomsbury Press, 2010, p. 13.

29. Reich, RB. Forward to Wilkinson, R, Pickett, K. *The Spirit Level: Why Greater Equality Makes Societies Stronger.* New York. Bloomsbury Press, 2010, p. ix.

30. Ibid # 28, p. 56.

31. Marmor, TR, Mashaw, JL, Pakutka, J. *Social Insurance: America's Neglected Heritage and Contested Future.* Los Angeles, CA. Sage Publications, 2014, pp. 219-220.

32. Nichols, J. McChesney, RW. Dollarocracy: The squabbling of Democrats and Republicans has become a sideshow to the theatre of plutocracy. *The Nation,* September 30, 2013.

33. Kuttner, R. The inequality puzzle. *The American Prospect,* March/April 2014, p. 5.

34. McIntyre, RS, Gardner, M, Phillips, R. *The Sorry State of Corporate Taxes: What Fortune 500 Firms Pay (or Don't Pay) in the USA and What They Pay Abroad—2008-2012.* Washington, D.C., February 2014.

35. Russolillo, S. Health stocks lead from the front. *Wall Street Journal,* March 31, 2014.

36. Meckler, L. How where we live deepens the nation's partisan split. *Wall Street Journal,* March 21, 2014: A1.

37. Livingston, A. Democrats facing political fallout on Medicare. *Roll Call,* April 1, 2014.

38. Nather, D. The Obamacare enthusiasm gap. *Politico,* March 31, 2014.

39. Lown, B. Physicians need to fight the business model of medicine. *Hippocrates* 12 (5): 25-28, 1998.

40. Woolhandler, S, Himmelstein, DU. When money is the mission—the high costs of investor-owned care. *New Engl J Med* 341: 444-446, 1999.

41. Mayer, C. Turning to the web to help pay medical bills. *Kaiser Health News*, July 2, 2013.

42. Marwick, C. Report: Health care reform must affirm "right." *JAMA* 270:1284-1285, 1993.

43. Churchill, L. *Rationing Health Care in America: Perceptions and Principles of Justice.* Notre Dame, IND. University of Notre Dame, 1987: 70-71, 90-91.

44. Light, DW. A conservative call for universal access to health care. *Penn Bioethics* 9 (4): 4-6, 2002.

CHAPTER 13

MYTHS AND MEMES AS BARRIERS TO HEALTH CARE REFORM

. . . For the great enemy of truth is very often not the lie—deliberate, contrived and dishonest—but the myth—persistent, persuasive, and unrealistic. Too often we hold fast to the clichés of our forebears. We subject all facts to a prefabricated set of interpretations. We enjoy the comfort of opinion without the discomfort of thought.

—John F. Kennedy, Commencement Address at
Yale University, June 11, 1962

Conflicting ideologies without facts have driven the debate over health care in this country for more than three decades, obscuring the real options for reform of our system. Lies and disinformation become established as myths. Then, when repeated enough over years, they can transform into memes, self-replicating ideas that are promulgated as "truths," without regard to their merits, and become accepted without question by much of our population. Unfortunately both myths and memes have been used for political purposes by opponents of reform to confuse the electorate and perpetuate problems in our market-based system.

This chapter has two goals: (1) to discuss myths and memes that have been used to support continuation of our present system; and (2) to describe those that have been intended to discredit the single-payer financing alternative.

MYTHS AND MEMES SUPPORTING THE
DEREGULATED PRIVATE MARKETPLACE

1. The free market will fix our system problems of access, costs and quality of health care.

This is a classic, ongoing myth, now a meme, that refuses to go away despite all the evidence refuting it for at least three decades. Earlier chapters make that case. We've tried the deregulated free market approach with all kinds of tweaks and patches—none have worked to contain health care costs or increase access, quality and efficiency of care. Yet the old, discredited market theory of health care lives on, as illustrated by this certain proclamation on the *Wall Street Journal's* Op-Ed page, by John Cochrane, professor of finance at the University of Chicago's Booth School of Business, about alternatives to Obamacare:

> *A much freer market in health care and health insurance can work, can deliver high quality, technically innovative care at much lower cost, and solve the pathologies of the pre-existing system.*[1]

> —John H. Cochrane, senior fellow of the Hoover Institution
> and adjunct scholar of the Cato Institute

Markets in health care just don't work the way they may in other industries or with other products. Kenneth Arrow, a leading economist at Columbia University, observed back in 1963 that uncertainty is the root cause of market failure in health care.[2] Patients have no way of knowing what care they will need, or when, while health professionals deal with uncertainty every day in clinical practice. Insurers deal with uncertainty by "experience rating" and medical underwriting to "lemon drop"—avoiding sicker patients—and "cherry pick"—selecting healthier patients for coverage.

There is much less competition in health care than market enthusiasts proclaim. Instead we have increasing consolidation of hospital systems and insurers, wide latitude to set prices to what the traffic will bear, and continued conflicts of interest that encourage wasteful, unnecessary and even harmful care.

It is surprising that most economists still buy the idea that competition in health care markets works to contain prices and provide more value than a more regulated market. They turn a blind eye to our own experience over three-plus decades, to international experience with health care systems, and even to luminaries in their own profession.

Dr. Friedrich A. Hayek, leading economist from the last century, who served as professor of social and moral sciences at the University of Chicago from 1950 to 1962 and was a co-recipient of the Nobel Memorial Prize in Economic Sciences in 1974, predicted the downsides of market capitalism as early as 1946:

Market capitalism will have the same inefficient, exploitative outcome as Soviet Communism if the ownership of resources becomes concentrated in the hands of fewer and fewer large corporations, and if economic business decisions come to be made by those relatively few individuals who own and/ or operate large concentrated corporations.[3]

We should have heeded Dr. Hayek's warnings almost 70 years ago, as earlier chapters have made clear. Instead what we have now is best described by Dr. Marcia Angell this way:

We've engaged in a massive and failed experiment in market-based medicine in the U.S. Rhetoric about the benefits of competition and profit-driven health care can no longer hide the reality: Our health system is in shambles.[4]

—Marcia Angell, M.D., former editor of *The New England Journal of Medicine* and author of *The Truth About Drug Companies: How They Deceive Us and What We Can Do About It.*

Despite the ongoing claims by market proponents that the "competitive marketplace" will contain health care costs, we have only to look at the last three decades to conclude that this is untrue. These five major reasons account for why deregulated markets can *never* succeed in controlling health care costs:

- There is little actual competition in health care markets.
- On the supply side, providers and suppliers have wide latitude to set prices.
- Our fragmented system does not allow for bulk purchasing.
- Our distorted reimbursement policies favor gaming of the system.
- Demand for health care is not as sensitive to prices as we might think.[5]

2. Private health insurance offers more choice and quality than a "one size fits all" government program.

In considering the possible merits of this statement, it is helpful to differentiate between two basic types of insurance. Mike Konzcai, fellow at the Roosevelt Institute, sees what we have in the private health insurance industry as a "neoliberal" approach, heavy on means-testing, private provisioning, and emphasis on choice and competition. The other basic type is public coverage through the federal government, such as traditional Medicare, with universal coverage of a defined set of benefits for all who qualify for them. Neoliberal insurance gives discretion to the states to help (or undermine) the process, segments the market, and is open to adverse selection. The public model is more efficient, reliable and offers higher value at lower cost.[6]

Yes, private insurance offers many choices, but for what coverage and at what cost? As we have seen, we get *less* coverage at higher cost, and with *less* reliability compared to traditional Medicare. The term "one size fits all" is used by market advocates to discredit the positives of universal coverage, playing on Americans' self-image of rugged individualism and independence. At the same time, most ordinary Americans are increasingly insecure about the costs of their health care and just one major illness or accident away from medical bankruptcy. As we saw in Chapter 3, Medicare coverage has been consistently rated more highly compared to private insurance.[7]

3. The U.S. has the best health care system in the world.

This is a common belief, fanned by conservatives and market advocates, that is more untrue than true. Though we are excellent in many parts of health care, other nations and systems are better than us in terms of access and quality of care for their populations. Despite many cross-national studies, many Americans still assume that we must be best since we have the latest technology and have so many specialists. In part, this thinking also reflects an attitude of American exceptionalism.

Here are some studies that show how far behind we are compared to many advanced countries around the world in terms of quality and outcomes of care:

- The U.S. has the worst record for preventable deaths among 19 Organization for Economic Cooperation and Development (OECD) countries; we also had the least improvement from 1997 to 2003 compared to those countries.[8]
- Longevity of Americans is less than that in many other countries that spend much less than we do on health care.[9]
- The U.S. ranks 42nd compared to other countries in deaths of children under five years of age.[10]
- The U.S. has one of the highest mortality rates in the world for dialysis patients[11], with rates 19 to 24 percent higher in the two largest for-profit dialysis chains than not-for-profit chains.[12]

Recall Figure 9.3 (page 159) that shows how poorly the U.S. compares with six other advanced countries in terms of overall system rankings for quality, access, efficiency, and equity of health care, as well as comparative rankings for living healthy, productive lives and per capita health expenditures.[13] And here are other studies that belie what we might think about the advantages of technology and numbers of specialists:

- Up to one-third of health care services in our market-based system are either inappropriate or unnecessary, and some actually harmful.[14]

- In areas of the country with more specialists, the quality of care is lower.[15]

4. Consumer-directed health care will contain health care costs.

This is the classic belief held by conservatives and most economists that patients will abuse any system when they don't have enough "skin in the game" through cost-sharing at the point of care. This was the whole idea behind the notion of Consumer-Driven Health Care (CDHC) that has permeated our system for many years. The assumption is that patients will overuse the system, especially if insured.

On the surface, this may seem to make sense, but its track record is quite different in practice. After three decades, CDHC has not been able to rein in continued inflation of health care costs. These are some arguments against the CDHC concept:

- Physicians, driven by a largely for-profit medical arms race, order most of the health care services that patients receive, and account for much more of the overuse of the system than patients do. Patients do not run to get a hip replacement unless they need it, even if insured.
- The more cost-sharing is imposed on patients with higher deductibles and co-payments, the more they forego timely and necessary care, resulting in *underuse* of care, as shown in Figure 13.1.[16]
- A 2004 RAND study found that doubling of co-payments led to less use of prescription drugs for diabetes and other chronic illness, together with a 17 percent increase in emergency room visits and a 10 percent increase in length of hospitalization.[17]
- Another study by RAND and the National Bureau of Economic Research found that increased cost-sharing is associated with increased use of ER visits, more hospitalizations, and worse clinical outcomes for patients with congestive heart failure, lipid disorders, diabetes, and schizophrenia.[18]

FIGURE 13.1

'Consumer Driven' Plans = Worse Access
Patients With High Deductibles Forego Needed Care

Patients Failing to Get Needed...

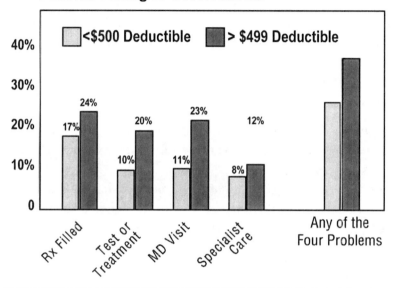

Source: Davis, K, Schoen, C, Stremikis, MPP. *Mirror, Mirror on the Wall: How the Performance of the U.S. Health System Compares Internationally.* New York. The Commonwealth Fund, 2010 update.
Reprinted with permission.

5. Everyone gets care anyhow through our current safety net.

Although this is widely believed, it is far from true, as my 2005 book, *Falling Through the Safety Net: Americans Without Health Insurance,* makes clear.[19] Yes, we do have the EMTALA law to provide emergency care for anyone, but this is not comprehensive, does not include follow-up care, and is increasingly expensive, especially as the numbers of free-standing private ERs grow. And yes, there is a loose patchwork of underfunded, mostly public programs, including community health centers and urgent care centers.

Much as many would like to deny and ignore, we have a

multi-tier, unfair system—based on ability to pay, not medical need—that denies access to adequate care to much of our population. A 2013 report from the Commonwealth Fund, *Health Care in the Two Americas: Findings from the Scorecard on State Health System Performance for Low-Income Populations*, shows how widespread health care disparities are in the U.S. This extensive report, the first to examine how well states' health care systems actually work, ranked states on 30 indicators, such as access to affordable care, preventive care, quality, and health outcomes. It found stark contrasts in access, quality and outcomes from state to state. As just two examples:

- Only 32 percent of low-income adults ages 50 or older received recommended preventive care, such as cancer screenings and vaccines.
- Asthma-related hospitalizations among children from low-income communities in New York were eight times higher than in Oregon, the state with the lowest rate.

Figure 13.2 illustrates these disparities by state.[20]

MYTHS AND MEMES THAT DISCREDIT SINGLE-PAYER

1. NHI is socialized medicine.

Conservative critics of NHI, joined of course by corporate stakeholders in our market-based system, are quick to call single-payer health insurance "socialized medicine." This is a fear strategy with a very long history. When President Truman advanced NHI in 1948, he did so with assurances to physicians, hospitals, and the public that delivery of care would continue in a private marketplace and that the government would only be involved in *financing* of that care. He kept emphasizing that this was in no way socialized medicine:

Socialized medicine means that all doctors are employees of the Government. The American people want no such system. No such system is here proposed.[21]

FIGURE 13.2

Two Americas: States' Health Systems
For Low-Income People

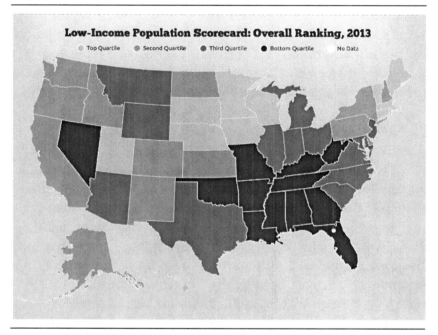

Source: Schoen, C, Radley, DC, Riley, P et al. Health Care in the Two Americas: Findings from the Scorecard on State Health System Performance for Low-Income Populations. *The Commonwealth Fund*, September 18, 2013.
Reprinted with permission

But organized medicine swiftly counter-attacked with this statement by Dr. Morris Fishbein, the AMA's president:

> *[This] is the first step toward the regimentation of utilities, of industry, of finance, and eventually of labor itself. This is the kind of regimentation that led to totalitarianism in Germany and the downfall of that nation . . . no one will ever convince the physicians of America that the . . . bill is not socialized medicine.*[22]

Critics on the right and stakeholders in our medical-industri-al complex use this approach whenever single-payer financing is raised, despite the fact that most other advanced countries around the world have universal health insurance, publicly financed in one way or another, with a private delivery system, as is the case in Canada. England is a true example of socialized medicine, with the government owning hospitals and other facilities and employ-ing physicians and other health professionals. However, as we have seen, it has a much better system in terms of access, costs, and quality for much less than we pay in this country.

2. NHI would be a government takeover.

This time-worn claim goes along with the alleged threat that single-payer national health insurance would bring socialized medicine. Opponents of the ACA have also attacked Obamacare as a broad overreach of government despite its many industry-friendly provisions favoring private markets. Hypocrisy and disinformation on the right seem to have no limits. Instead of a government takeover, Tom Scully, former administrator of CMS during the George W. Bush administration, had it correct when he told an audience hosted by the Potomac Research Group, a Belt-way firm that advises large investors on government policy, that the ACA is more capitalistic than anything we've seen to date and will make some people very rich.[23] Wall Street agrees, as shown by health care stocks soaring by almost 40 percent in 2013, the highest of any sector in the S & P 500.[24]

As we shall see in the next chapter, NHI will simplify the *financing* of health care, but leave the *delivery* system in private hands in a more efficient system available to all Americans. Phy-sicians, other health care professionals, hospitals, other facilities, the drug and medical device industries, and other parts of the sys-tem will continue to compete on the basis of the availability and quality of their services and products in an expanded market of 310 million people.

3. We can't afford NHI—it would break the bank.

The assumption for this myth is that patients will overuse health care if they gain access to care without any cost-sharing as in single-payer financing. This is the conceptual lynchpin of consumer-directed health care, which has failed over so many years to rein in costs. The foregoing chapters give clear evidence that this concept does not work, and instead leads many patients to forego essential care because of costs, usually involving increased health care costs down the road. As just one example of this problem, one in four uninsured cancer patients delay or forego care because of costs.[25]

As we saw in the last chapter, what we *cannot* afford is the present unaccountable system with uncontrollable prices and costs. Overutilization of health care is indeed a huge problem and cause of soaring health care costs, but it is not about patients abusing the system. The real causes of health care inflation range from technological advances, changing thresholds for defining "disease", increasing prevalence of chronic disease in an aging population, and wasteful administrative costs in an inefficient system, to corporate profiteering throughout the medical-industrial complex and *physician*-induced demand, since physicians order most health care services that are delivered.

Canada's experience in launching its universal single-payer system in the 1970s gives us a data point supporting the premise that patients will not abuse such a system and that total health care costs can be controlled by single-payer financing. Instead of a rush to unnecessary care, Canadians began receiving mostly necessary care, much that had been delayed, and their system has consistently provided better health outcomes ever since at just one-half of what the U.S. spends on health care.[26]

4. NHI would ration care.

Rationing, the feared R word, is trotted out by most opponents of single-payer as if NHI would limit health care more than it already is in our ability-to-pay system. This, of course, is the opposite of what will happen with NHI—all Americans will, for the first time, have access to all necessary and appropriate care with free choice of physician and hospital anywhere in the country. Yes, we should then also have a national, science-based institute with the expertise and authority to assess what services and procedures offer enough benefit to be covered.

All health care systems ration care in one way or another. Our present system rations by willingness and ability to pay, not by what services or procedures are necessary, appropriate or cost-effective. Our present approach for the approval of new prescription drugs, for example, falls far short of the kind of scientific rigor we should expect in terms of efficacy and cost-effectiveness. The approval process through the FDA involves advisory committees with members frequently having conflicts of interest with drug manufacturers, together with other industry-friendly provisions as described in Dr. Marcia Angell's excellent book, *The Truth About the Drug Companies: How They Deceive Us and What To Do About It*. Examples abound that cry out for a more rigorous evidence-based approach, such as that used by the National Institute for Health and Clinical Excellence (NICE) in the United Kingdom. These examples show how loose the approval process is in this country:

- Lacking clinical evidence that a 23 mg dose of the Alzheimer's drug Aricept is more effective than a 10 mg dose (and that efficacy is open to some question), the FDA approved the larger dose even though patients stopped taking the larger dose twice as often as the 10 mg dose due to adverse side effects.[27]
- Johnson & Johnson's A.S.R., a metal artificial hip replacement, received expedited FDA review and approval without clinical trials. But the devices had a high failure rate, disabling many patients with pain, often requiring removal. It was finally recalled by the company, but only after achieving a market share of almost one-third of an estimated 250,000 hip replacements annually in the U.S.[28]

5. NHI would stifle innovation.

This rhetoric from free market advocates has been repeated for many years whenever a new government program is being discussed, no matter how friendly to industry. A current example is this statement by Sally Pipes, president and CEO of the Pacific Research Institute, a right-wing think tank, about the threat to innovation posed by the ACA:

We are going to see a tremendous decline in research and development and the funding needed to develop new drugs. We are taking a step backwards in our ability to develop life-extending drugs.[29]

The real story, of course, is that the pharmaceutical industry has been the most profitable of all industries for many years, thriving through the largesse of government policies that include ongoing basic science research by the National Institutes of Health and various tax credits for post-FDA marketing research by drug companies. Markets have been expanded by the Medicare Prescription Drug, Improvement and Modernization Act of 2003 (MMA) as well as by the ACA, all the while leaving the industry with wide latitude to set its own prices. The Pharmaceutical Research and Manufacturers of America (PhRMA), the drug industry's powerful trade group, has lobbied successfully over the years to prevent importation of drugs from other countries and avoid bulk purchasing of drugs as the Veterans Administration does in discounting prices by more than 40 percent.

Meanwhile, we do not hear inconvenient truths about innovation in the drug industry. Two-thirds of new drug applications to the FDA each year are just reformulations or minor modifications of existing drugs or requests for new uses.[30] Many are "me-too" drugs being marketed as "new." A large percentage of breakthrough drugs are developed in Europe and other countries. And PhRMA consistently exaggerates its R & D costs, most of which are in the marketing phase with little scientific rigor, and represent little more than one-third of what the industry spends on marketing and administration.[31]

6. NHI would lead to excess bureaucracy.

This myth, though widely perceived by many, is absurd on its face, especially when one considers the extreme bureaucracy that we tolerate now in trying to keep an obsolete private health insurance industry alive through government subsidies and industry-friendly contortions. Recall Figure 2.1 (page 26), which shows the exponential growth in numbers of administrators since 1990 compared to the numbers of physicians. Now consider just one part of the ACA—the exchanges—and we can get some idea of the added complexity of trying to figure out what comparative costs, coverage, and eligibility requirements might apply as people go to the exchanges for help in navigating the new "system." (Figure 13.3)

With single-payer national health insurance, administration would be simplified, everyone is covered for a comprehensive set of benefits, there is no cost-sharing, and overhead would likely be less than 3 or 4 percent (that of traditional Medicare already is just 1.5 or 2 percent).

Comparisons with our single-payer neighbor to the North reveal just how burdensome our bureaucracy is now, aggravated as it is by the ACA. Physicians' billing and office expenses in this country are almost four times that of their counterparts in Canada. U.S. physicians are finding that their paperwork is increasing all the time, despite their growing use of electronic health records, with more than one in four physicians spending more than 15 hours a week on paperwork.[32]

7. Canada's experience with single-payer shows how it won't work here.

Opponents of single-payer NHI are quick to point out the alleged problems of the Canadian system in derogatory terms— if not claiming it as socialized, which it is not, then hobbled by

FIGURE 13.3

Exchange Functions
Under the ACA

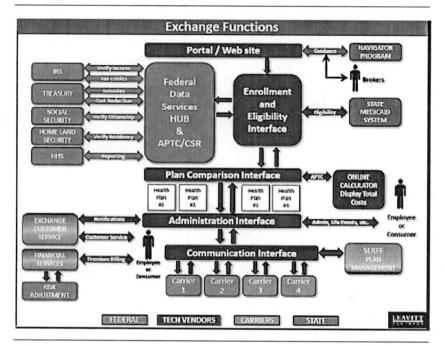

Source: The National Health Program Slide-Show Guide. Physicians for a National Health Program. Chicago, IL, September 11, 2013

long wait times. They do so out of ignorance of the many strong points of the Canadian system as well as outright disinformation intended to perpetuate corporate stakeholders' grip on our deregulated marketplace.

For openers, the Canadian system beats the U.S. system hands down on measures of access, cost containment, affordability, equity, quality and outcomes of care, as shown by results of cross-national studies mentioned earlier. Cost containment, since the enactment of Canada's national health program is particularly striking in comparison with health care costs in our two countries since 1960 (Figure 13.4).

Even more impressive is the difference in Medicare spending per senior in the U.S. and Canada, which has been about three

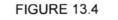

FIGURE 13.4

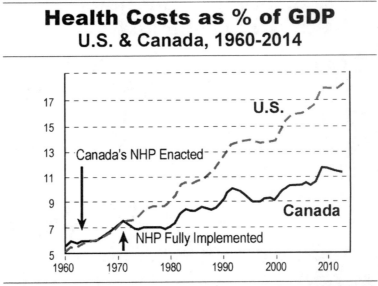

Health Costs as % of GDP
U.S. & Canada, 1960-2014

Source: Statistics Canada, Canadian Institute for Health Info & NCHS/Commerce Dept.

times higher in the U.S. over the last 25 years. This is no accident. With its single-payer system, coupled with a private delivery system, Canada is able to keep administrative costs low (16.7 percent of health care spending vs. 31 percent in the U.S.), while employing lump-sum global budgets for hospitals, controlling capital expenditures, bulk purchasing for drugs and medical devices, emphasizing primary care, and excluding private insurers. All of that while providing universal comprehensive coverage with full choice of physician and hospital.[33]

Opponents of the Canadian system on this side of the border have some evidence on their side when it comes to waiting times, but again that issue is blown out of proportion, especially with inaccurate and misleading reports from the right-wing Frazier Institute. They typically cite delays in getting an MRI or elective surgery.[34] But to be fair, remember that Canada spends just one-half of what the U.S. spends on health care, and that lower-income Americans, even those newly insured on Medicaid through the ACA, may have great difficulty in finding *any* physician to see them and may wait for months or indefinitely to see specialists. Over the last ten years, Canada has made excellent progress in cutting wait times in five priority clinical areas—cancer, heart, diagnostic imaging, joint replacement, and sight restoration.[35]

CONCLUSION

We have covered a lot of ground in this chapter in an attempt to explain and debunk many myths and memes that unfortunately remain part of our national debate over the future of U.S. health care, despite their lack of merit. Mostly they still miss the fundamentals of the debate, such as who is the health care system for—patients and families or profiteering corporate interests? We still need to cut through the thicket of deception and disinformation to get to the basics. This observation by Robert Kuttner, whom we met in the last chapter and author of the 2007 book, *The Squandering of America: How the Failure of Our Politics Undermines Our Prosperity*, is right on target:

> *Going forward, leaders would do well to articulate a few bold, clear ideas that identify them with the economic frustrations and aspirations of citizens—and along the way to rehabilitate the idea of public remedy. Instead of programs of byzantine complexity to fill in the gaps in private health insurance without frightening the health insurance industry or the Business Roundtable, why not support a proven idea that can be summed up in three easy words—"Medicare for all"—and dare private industry and the Republicans to oppose it?*[36]

References

1. Cochrane, JH. What to do when Obamacare unravels. *Wall Street Journal*, December 26, 2013: A13.
2. Arrow, KJ. Uncertainty and the welfare economics of medical care. *American Economic Review* 53: 941-973, 1963.

3. Hayek, FA. *American Economic Review*, 1946.
4. Angell, M. Sweeping health care reform proposed by nation's top physicians. Press release. Physicians for a National Health Program. Chicago, May 1, 2001.
5. Geyman, JP. Market mythology in health care: Why markets can never control health care costs. *Huffington Post*, September 16, 2008.
6. Konzcai, M. What kind of problem is the ACA rollout for liberalism? Next New Deal, *The blog of the Roosevelt Institute*, October 23, 2013.
7. Davis, K, Schoen, C, Doty, M et al. Medicare versus private insurance: rhetoric and reality. *Health Affairs Web Exclusive* W 321, October 9, 2002.
8. Nolte, E, McKee, CM. Measuring the health of nations: Updating an earlier analysis. *Health Affairs* 28 (1): 63, 2008.
9. UC Atlas of Global Inequality, Health Care Spending: Large Differences, Unequal Results, November 15, 2007. Available at ucatlas.ucsc.edu/spend.php
10. Rajaratnam, JK, Marcus, JR, Flaxman, AD et al. Neonatal, postnatal, childhood and under-5 mortality for 187 countries, 1970-2010: A systematic analysis of progress towards Millennium Development Goal 4. *The Lancet* 375: 1888-2008, 2010.
11. Fields, R. In dialysis, life-saving care at great risk and cost. *ProPublica*, November 9, 2010.
12. Zhang, Y, Cotter DJ, Thamer, M. The effect of dialysis claims on mortality among patients receiving dialysis. *Health Services Research* 46 (3): 747-767, 2011.
13. Davis, K, Schoen, C, Stremikis, MPP. Mirror, mirror on the wall: How the performance of the U.S. health system compares internationally. New York. *The Commonwealth Fund*, 2010 update.
14. Wennberg, JB, Fisher, ES, Skinner, JS. Geography and the debate over Medicare reform. *Health Affairs Web Exclusive* W-103, February 13, 2002.
15. Ibid # 14.
16. Davis, K. Half of insured adults with high-deductible health plans experience medical bill or debt problems. New York. *The Commonwealth Fund*, January 27, 2005.
17. Goldman, DP et al. Pharmacy benefits and the use of drugs by the chronically ill. *JAMA* 291: 2344-2350, 2004.
18. Goldman, DP, Joyce, GF, Zheng, Y. Prescription drug cost-sharing: Association with medication and medical utilization and spending and health. *JAMA* 298 (11): 61-88, 2007.
19. Geyman, JP. *Falling Through the Safety Net: Americans Without Health Insurance*. Monroe, ME. Common Courage Press, 2005.
20. Schoen, C, Radley, DC, Riley, P et al. *Health Care in the Two Americas: Findings from the Scorecard on State Health System Performance for Low-Income Populations*, The Commonwealth Fund, September 18, 2013.
21. Truman, HS. *Special Message to the Congress Recommending a Comprehensive Health Program*, November 19, 1945. http://www.trumanlibrary.org/publicpapers/index.php?pid=483
22. Fishbein, M. Quoted in "Fishbein assails new health plan, Truman's national program condemned as 'socialized medicine' at its worst". *New York Times*, November 27, 1945.
23. Davidson, A. The President wants you to get rich on Obamacare. *The New York Times Magazine*, October 30, 2013.

24. Soltas, E. Nobody should get rich off Obamacare. *Bloomberg View*, December 3, 2013.
25. Wolfe, SM. Outrage of the month! 50 million uninsured in the U.S. equals 50,000+ avoidable deaths each year. *Health Letter* 28 (1): 11, January 2012.
26. Armstrong, P, Armstrong, H, Fegan, C. *Universal Health Care: What the United States Can Learn from the Canadian Experience*. New York. The New Press. 1998, pp. 131-132.
27. Holzer, B. FDA ignores negative feedback on Alzheimer's drug Aricept. *Public Citizen News* 31 (4): 20, 2011.
28. Meier, B. Metal hips failing fast, report says. *New York Times*, September 16, 2011: B1.
29. Pipes, S. As quoted by Duncan, J. Obamacare's deadly side effect. *Newsmax*, December 2013, p. 12.
30. Field, RI. *Mother of Invention: How the Government Created Free-Market Health Care*. New York. Oxford University Press, 2014, p. 51.
31. Angell, M. *The Truth about Drug Companies: How They Deceive Us and What We Can Do About It*. New York. Random House, 2004.
32. Medscape Physician Compensation Report, 2012, 2013.
33. Himmelstein, DU. Woolhandler, S. Cost control in a parallel universe: Medicare spending in the United States and Canada. *Arch Int Med* 172 (22): 1764-1766, 2012.
34. McCanne, D. Comment in Quote of the Day, "42,000 Canadians come to the United States for care" — Really? March 17, 2014. Available at quote-of-the-day@mccanne.org
35. Canadian Institute for Health Information (CIHI). *Wait Times for Priority Procedures in Canada, 2014.* March 2014.
36. Kuttner, R. *The Squandering of America: How the Failure of Our Politics Undermines Our Prosperity.* New York. Alfred Knopf, 2010, p. 300.

CHAPTER 14

WHAT WILL SINGLE-PAYER HEALTH CARE LOOK LIKE?

So long as private, for-profit companies handle the insurance, and so long as physicians and hospitals are driven by income-maximizing incentives that reward inefficiency and overutilization of resources, rising costs will continue to be at the center of our health care problem.[1]

—Arnold S. Relman, M.D., former editor of *The New England Journal of Medicine* and author of *A Second Opinion: Rescuing America's Health Care*

Despite all the fears, change will come. The market system is a devastating failure, and nearly every major public opinion poll finds health care at or near the top of Americans' concerns. . . . Ultimately, the driving forces behind change will come from two sources: working Americans who are disenchanted with ever-rising costs and shrinking care, and U.S. corporations, which are increasingly refusing to pick up the added costs.[2]

—Donald L Bartlett and James B Steele, investigative reporters, at-large editors at *Time*, and authors of *Critical Condition: How Health Care in America Became Big Business—and Bad Medicine.*

It is now time to describe what a single-payer system of financing U.S. health care will look like when it does happen, which is inevitable given the downward course of all market-based incremental tweaks. This chapter has three goals: (1) to summarize the key features of single-payer national health insurance (NHI); (2) to briefly discuss frequently asked questions about NHI; and (3) to consider winners and losers of this change.

KEY FEATURES OF SINGLE-PAYER NHI

This is neither a new nor fringe concept, having been developed over the past 25 years, especially through the leadership and writings of Physicians for a National Health Program (PNHP), founded in 1989 with a current membership of more than 19,000 U.S. physicians. Drawing from the research and writings of its leaders over the years, these are some of its key features.[3,4]

Universal access to comprehensive coverage

Universal coverage of all Americans is assured for necessary health care, in a one-class single risk pool, portable from state to state, regardless of patients' age or ability to pay. Patients seeing their providers just present their NHI cards at the point of service. Today's widespread confusion over changing coverage requirements of the ACA will go away.[5]

No out-of-pocket payments

Out-of-pocket payments are eliminated, since co-payments and deductibles are financial barriers to care and have not worked over many years to contain health care costs. All costs of covered care are covered by NHI without billing to patients.

Free choice of physician, other providers, hospital, and other facilities

With free choice there are no longer narrow networks or private insurers telling you who or where to go for care. No more listening to that first question—"Do you have insurance, and what is it?" Your NHI card is all you need when you need care. Continuity of care with providers of choice will be much improved with single-payer financing.

A defined set of benefits

Coverage includes all standard medical care, including all physician and hospital care, outpatient care, dental services, vision services, rehabilitation, long-term care, home care, mental health care, and prescription drugs. A national, tax-funded health care coverage plan will be prevented by the U.S. Constitution from restricting any services based on religious beliefs, as was brought into question by the recent Hobby Lobby decision of the U.S. Supreme Court.[6]

Financing

The program is paid for by combining current sources of government health spending into a single fund with modest progressive taxes that will end up with 95 percent of Americans paying less than what they now pay for insurance premiums, deductibles, co-payments, actual care, and out-of-pocket payments (see Figure 12.1 on page 205).

Effective cost controls

Coverage for all Americans for all necessary health care is made possible, *without any increase in total health care spending,* by cost controls that include negotiated annual budgets to hospitals and other facilities, negotiated fees with physicians and other providers, transition to a not-for-profit system, and bulk purchasing of prescription drugs (as the Veterans Administration has been doing for many years with 40 percent discounts). Large savings, estimated at $592 billion annually, will be achieved through simplified administration, in largest part by eliminating administrative waste of the private health insurance industry ($476 billion each year). These savings can reduce the deficit by $154 billion in the first year, as we saw in Chapter 12. Additional savings will be realized by eliminating about one-half of the 30 percent of hospital budgets that now go for billing and administration.[7]

Transition to not-for-profit health care facilities and providers

Because the for-profit business "ethic" diverts resources from patient care to investors, and profit-driven incentives distort the delivery and quality of care, single-payer financing will transition to a not-for-profit service ethic. H.R. 676 includes funding to absorb the cost of converting investor-owned health care facilities to non-profit status spread out over a 15-year transition period. Owners of investor-owned facilities will not be compensated for loss of business opportunities or for administrative capacity not used by NHI.

National scientific body for ongoing assessment of evidence for and against treatments in health care

This body should be protected from political interference and have the authority to make coverage decisions about the efficacy and cost-effectiveness of comparative approaches to preventive care as well as diagnosis and treatment of disease. The goal will be to cover treatments that make a difference for both individuals and the population at large. Inappropriate, unnecessary and harmful services will not be covered. Assessments will be transparent and based on best science and the public interest.

Clinical decision-making

Clinical decision-making will be between the physician or other provider and the patient, respecting the patient's autonomy. Denial of necessary services by insurers or employers will be a thing of the past.

Health care system planning

Health planning will be strengthened to improve the availability of resources and minimize wasteful duplication. The NHI program will fund the purchase of expensive equipment, capital improvements, and new construction of needed facilities through regional health planning boards. Investor-owned facilities will be phased out over a period of years. Investor-owned facilities, including hospitals, nursing homes, HMOs and clinics, will be compensated by the NHI program for the loss of their clinical facilities, as well as any computers and administrative facilities used to manage NHI.

Public accountability, not corporate dictates

Today's confusion and lack of transparency empowers insurers and employers to pursue their financial interests with little regard for the patient. Too many health care decisions are now made behind closed corporate doors. This will be replaced with an open transparent process that determines coverage decisions based on scientific evidence and the public interest.

FREQUENTLY ASKED QUESTIONS [8]

1. *How can we afford a system wherein everyone has access to all necessary health care?*

Cost savings, estimated at $592 billion annually, will go a long way in expanding universal access to our entire population. Administrative simplification with single-payer will eliminate most of the more than 30 percent of the wasteful administrative costs in our current multi-payer system. NHI will allow people to seek care for illness and injuries from any licensed health care provider without financial barriers, which can permit earlier diagnosis and more effective treatment of many conditions. In the long run, costs can be controlled and made affordable system-wide by improved health planning, elimination of unnecessary duplication, negotiated fees and budgets, and investment in procedures and services that work and are cost-effective.

2. How can over-utilization of care be avoided?

As discussed in the last chapter, the largest driver of current over-utilization of health services in this country is *physician-induced* demand, not patients abusing the system. As NHI makes the transition to a service-oriented not-for-profit system, perverse profit incentives that now encourage providers to deliver inappropriate and unnecessary procedures and services will go away. Other countries have found that utilization of health care does indeed increase, at least in the short term, when systems of universal care are introduced, but that most of the care was necessary and often previously delayed or foregone.

3. *This sounds like pie in the sky; how can we be sure it will work?*

All we have to do is look at the long-term experience of almost all industrialized countries around the world. Yes, they have variations to their approach to universal care, but most have cost controls in place with either single-payer or highly regulated, more accountable insurers. Western Europe, Scandinavia, the United Kingdom, Australia, New Zealand, Taiwan and other countries spend little more than one-half what we spend on health care and get better health outcomes for their populations. Our American "exceptionalism" as a health care system is marked by the extent of how wasteful and expensive our system is.

4. *What will happen to quality of care?*

This can only improve as all Americans gain early access to all necessary health care. Today, despite some gains in access through the ACA, many millions of Americans remain uninsured and we still have an epidemic of underinsurance. Since single-payer provides equal access to care for everyone regardless of age, income, employment or diagnosis, all Americans have access to available resources within a one-class system. Continuity of medical and nursing care will be improved. Health care professionals can spend more of their time on direct patient care with few administrative hassles and assured payment of reasonable fees. Preventive care and evidence-based screening will be available for individuals and populations, with an increased priority for public health. Electronic health records will become more standardized to facilitate monitoring of quality of care and patient outcomes with more emphasis on continuous quality improvement.[9]

5. *Do we have a strong enough primary care sector to make this work?*

The primary care shortage is a major problem, and will be in the early years of NHI, since primary care is already stretched thin. As we have seen in earlier chapters, our largely for-profit market-based system favors the more procedure-oriented, higher paid specialties, which has led to the long-standing imbalance between the primary care specialties and other specialties in the U.S. Countries with best-performing systems have at least one-half of their physicians in generalist primary care practice—about 70 percent in the UK and 50 percent in Canada. Financing reform under NHI will decrease the disparity of physician payment by specialty and make primary care a more attractive career choice for graduating medical students seeking a chance to make a difference. We are already seeing promising directions to stabilize and enhance primary care practice, including patient-centered medical homes and organized team practice. Other useful approaches that can be enabled by NHI include reimbursement reform, loan forgiveness programs for graduating medical students entering primary care residencies, increased funding for primary care residencies, and reallocation of graduate medical education training slots by specialty.[10]

6. *Won't I pay more taxes with NHI?*

Many are not aware that about 60 percent of today's health care system is already financed by public money—federal and state taxes, property taxes, and tax subsidies, especially to employers to help pay for their employees' health insurance. Private employers pay about 21 percent of health care costs, while individuals pay the rest for premiums, deductibles, co-payments and out-of-pocket costs. This is a regressive way to finance health care, with middle and lower-income people paying a much higher percentage of their income for health care than do people with higher incomes.

With NHI, public funds designated for Medicare and Medicaid will be re-directed to NHI, together with new progressive taxes as outlined in Chapter 12 (Table 12.1) (Page 205)[11] As we have seen, 95 percent of us will pay less tax than we are now paying when NHI is enacted. Table 14.1 shows how household incomes will be affected at four different annual income levels from $25,000 to $500,000 by new progressive taxes funding NHI. We can see that households with incomes of $25,000 and $50,000 will save 18.8 and 13.9 percent of their incomes, respectively, while none will pay more until their incomes exceed $225,000 per year.[12]

TABLE 14.1

IMPACT OF NHI TAXES ON HOUSEHOLD INCOMES

Gross income level	$25,000	$53,000	$225,000	$500,000
Payroll taxes				
3% on below $53,000	$366	$956	$1,590	$1,590
6% on above $53,000			$1,896	$4,680
Income Surtax				
6% high income, above $225,000				$26,340
6% all unearned income	$108	$165	$5,771	$17,850
Tobin tax on stock transfers	$253	$372	$10,243	$39,788
Total	$727	$1,493	$19,500	$90,248
Share of gross income	2.9%	2.8%	8.7%	18.0%
Current health care share(with imputed taxes)	22.7%	17.3%	12.7%	10.5%
Remaining out-of-pocket as share of income	2.0%	0.7%	0.1%	0.0%
Change in income with HR 676 as share of gross income	18.8%	13.9%	3.9%	-7.6%

Note: Payroll taxes are assessed only on the wage panel income. The 6% tax rate is assessed on wage income above $53,000. The 6% high income surtax is assessed on income other than income from pensions and transfers (income and in-kind). The 6% income surtax on unearned income is assessed on income from dividends, profits, interest, and capital gains. The Tobin tax share is estimated by allocating the expected revenue across income groups according to their share of total stock holdings. Current health share is estimated from Ketsche (Ketsche et al. 2011) updated to 2013 by increasing health spending at the national rate.

Source: Friedman, G. Personal communication, January 26, 2014.

7. *Will health care be rationed under NHI?*

We already ration care in our present system—in a cruel way based on ability to pay, not medical need. We also ration care in the ways that we set health policy. As a recent example, the states that have decided not to expand Medicaid under the ACA have denied care to many Americans who remain uninsured. A recent study estimates that at least 7,100 people will die without this Medicaid coverage.[13] Today's rationing is unnecessary, since we already have plenty of money in the system to afford NHI.

All health care systems ration care in one way or another, since there are never enough resources available to meet every need. The point is to do the best for the most with resources available.

8. *Will there be less competition in a NHI system?*

We have seen in earlier chapters how today's competition between hospitals, insurers and other corporate interests in our medical-industrial complex is about market share and profits and returns to shareholders, not primarily about providing service to patients. Contrary to the continued claims by advocates of "free markets", this kind of "competition" does not hold down costs. Instead it is wasteful, expensive, and inefficient, and is itself a major driver of uncontrolled inflation of health care costs.

That environment will change under NHI, when physicians, other providers, hospitals and other facilities will compete for patients based on quality of care and dedication to service—the old-fashioned way. Drug companies will have to compete based on the efficacy and cost-effectiveness of their drugs, not by the persuasiveness of their advertising and marketing.

9. *Will there be any role for private health insurance?*

The private insurance industry as we know it today will be eliminated under NHI. All Americans have to be included in a single risk pool in order to provide universal coverage and contain costs in a sustainable way. The comprehensive benefits package with NHI will eliminate the need for supplemental coverage. Whatever role private insurers may have in the future, they will not be permitted to duplicate the same benefits as the NHI program.

10. *What will happen to those employed by private insurers?*

Although the new NHI system will still need people to administer claims, administration will shrink substantially. The new system will no longer need the many jobs that are now involved in billing, eligibility determination, and advertising. Hospitals, clinics, nursing homes and other facilities will need fewer administrative staff. At the same time, there will be a greater need for staff in the fields of long-term care, home health care, and public health. Many employees of private insurers can be retrained to enter these and related fields. The budget of H.R. 676 includes the cost of unemployment insurance and retraining of displaced insurance and provider administrative personnel.

11. *Is ERISA a barrier in the way NHI is implemented?*

ERISA (the Employees Retirement Income Security Act) prevents a state from requiring that a self-insured employer provide certain benefits to their employees. But NHI will replace employer-sponsored insurance with a new Medicare for all system with states then requiring employers to pay a payroll tax into the new health care trust fund, clearly a legal change.

12. *Won't this be just another huge bureaucracy?*

By no means. The private insurance industry is already a massive bureaucracy involved largely in cherry-picking healthier people, avoiding sicker people, denying claims, and maximizing profits. Its medical loss ratio (what it *doesn't* pay for actual health care) ranges from 15 to 20 percent. No longer will we have thousands of private insurance plans, each with its own paperwork, enrollment, premiums, marketing, rules and regulations. Contrast that with traditional Medicare's overhead of about two percent. Even if NHI gets its administrative overhead down below five percent, that will be an enormous gain in efficiency and cost savings.

13. *Who will run the NHI system?*

There will be a single insurance plan across the country, administered by public or quasi-public agencies with elected and appointed members representing the public. These national agencies will decide on what is covered and negotiate physician fees and hospital budgets, with transparency and accountability to the public interest. A national agency (yet to be named) will evaluate the merits of new technologies and make coverage decisions. State agencies will assess community needs and make health planning decisions about needs for facilities and expensive equipment. Clinical decisions remain in the hands of patients and their health care professionals, as they should.

14. *Why not allow the wealthy to buy their own care outside of the NHI system?*

The strength, efficiency and fairness of NHI depends on the inclusion of all Americans in the best system that the country can afford, eliminating our current and past discrimination based on class and ability to pay. The NHI program will be weakened if the wealthy are permitted to jump the queue and get the same benefits as NHI under a private plan. We know from the experience of other countries that growth of private care in parallel with the public system creates a lobby for underfunding the public system. On the other hand, when the wealthy are required to use the NHI program, if they are dissatisfied, they will use their political influence to advocate for improvements in the public program, to the benefit of all.

15. What will happen to the costs of malpractice liability insurance with NHI?

These costs, for several reasons, will drop markedly with NHI. First, about one-half of all malpractice awards go to pay present and future medical costs, such as for infants born with serious disabilities. NHI will eliminate the need for these awards. Second, many malpractice awards result from a lack of continuity of care and miscommunication between physicians and patients. Our present system is increasingly fragmented with restricted choice of physicians and providers, a problem not resolved by electronic health record systems that don't communicate well with each other. NHI will restore full choice of physician and providers, leading to improved continuity and trust in care. Third, we know that the single-payer systems can be harnessed to improve quality and reduce costs of malpractice liability insurance.[14-16]

WINNERS AND LOSERS WITH NHI

NHI will be an enormous step ahead for our society. It is completely in step with traditional American values, including efficiency, choice, value, equity and integrity. These values have been long-standing and are echoed by both major political parties. NHI will bring Americans together around health care as a right, as it is in most other advanced countries around the world, instead of a privilege based on ability to pay. Many millions of uninsured and underinsured will gain access to care and their outcomes will improve. NHI will especially help to alleviate the current crisis in mental health care, since only about one-quarter of those with serious mental illness have any form of private insurance.[17] NHI can also bring a greater sense of social solidarity and help to narrow the widening inequality gap in the country.

Table 14.2 compares the differences in values between single-payer and multi-payer financing systems for health care.[18]

TABLE 14.2

Alternative Financing Systems and American Values

TRADITIONAL VALUE	Single-Payer	Multi-Payer
Efficiency	↑	↓
Choice	↑	↓
Affordability	↑	↓
Actuarial value	↑	↓
Fiscal responsibility	↑	↓
Equitable	↑	↓
Accountable	↑	↓
Integrity	↑	↓
Sustainable	↑	↓

Source: Geyman, JP. *Health Care Wars: How Market Ideology and Corporate Power Are Killing Americans.* Friday Harbor, WA. Copernicus Healthcare, 2012, p. 198.

Most win with NHI—first and most important, the *raison d'etre* of any health care system—patients and their families, all 310 million Americans. With just one structural change in financing, they immediately gain access to all necessary health care, with full choice of physician and hospital, and with portable reliable coverage throughout the country. They pay into the system through progressive taxes based on an equitable basis. NHI joins with Social Security as a bedrock of society. We move toward a not-for-profit service-oriented system with increased public accountability and elimination of profiteering. Compared to the byzantine complexity and fragmentation of the ACA, the new system will be easy for patients to navigate.

Business and labor join the winners' circle. Employers will pay less than they do now for health care, and will be relieved of the burden of providing employer-sponsored health insurance. Small businesses will no longer face the prospects of being kicked off group coverage under the ACA's definition of "employer", have to search for other coverage, or face fines.[19] Business will gain a healthier workforce and be better able to compete in a global economy with countries whose systems provide universal access to health care. Walter Reuther, as national president of the United Auto Workers more than 50 years ago, saw this day coming:

When American corporations reached the point where they couldn't make their business more efficient without making it less profitable, when their dependency ratios soared to unimaginable heights, when they got tens of billions behind in their health-care obligations, when the cost of carrying thousands of retirees forced them to stare bankruptcy in the face, they would come around to the idea that markets work best when the burdens of benefits are broadly shared.[20]

Hospitals, clinics, community health centers, nursing homes and other facilities will gain predictable negotiated annual budgets with administrative simplification. They will gain respect from the public as they shift away from profits to a service ethic.

Physicians and other health professionals will be freed from their daily hassles and paperwork in dealing with today's requirements of multiple insurers with different drug formularies. Physicians now spend an average of one-sixth of their working hours on administration.[21] They will be able to spend most of their time in direct patient care, and no longer have to deal with second-guessing and denial of services by insurance bureaucrats. We can expect that primary care and other shortage specialties will be better reimbursed, while some specialized procedures and services, now over-reimbursed, will receive less. Since all patients will be insured, payments will be assured, overhead markedly reduced, and losses due to charity care a thing of the past.

A recent study of historical polling data from 1966 through 2014 has documented erosion of the public trust in the leaders of the medical profession from 73 percent in 1966 to only 34 percent now. Moreover, just 23 percent of the public express a great deal or quite a bit of confidence in our health care system.[22] With NHI, we can anticipate that the public's trust in medicine and the health care system will be restored, together with increased career satisfaction among physicians.

The biggest loser when NHI is enacted, of course, will be the private insurance industry, but it has had a long run and has priced itself out of the market for many years. It should not be bailed out because of its size and political power, as the ACA has done. The huge compensation packages of its CEOs will disappear, but many workers in the industry can be retrained for new roles with the NHI.

Other losers under NHI include the drug, medical device, medical supply, and other health-related industries that lose their present latitude to set their own prices and have to deal with deep discounts through monopsony purchasing by the government. Their shareholders and Wall Street will have to adapt to a former medical-industrial complex in transition to a not-for-profit service industry. Many administrative and marketing jobs in today's private health sector will disappear. Today's profiteering by hospitals, physicians and other providers will be reined in to a more accountable system as today's market-driven inappropriate and unnecessary care is squeezed out of the system.

Given the long history of failed health care reform over the years and the enormous size and political clout of the corporate stakeholders in our medical-industrial complex that soaks up almost one-fifth of our GDP, is there any chance that NHI can finally be enacted in this country? That becomes the subject of the next and last chapter.

References

1. Relman, AS, *A Second Opinion: Rescuing America's Health Care*. New York. Public Affairs, A Century Foundation Book, 2007, p. 139.
2. Bartlett, DL. Steele, JB. *Critical Condition: How Health Care in America Became Big Business—and Bad Medicine.* New York. Doubleday, 2004, pp. 248-249.
3. The Physicians' Working Group for Single-Payer National Health Insurance. *JAMA* 290 (6): 798-805, 2003.
4. Himmelstein, DU, Woolhandler, S. National health insurance or incremental reform: aim high, or at our feet. *Amer. J Public Health* 93: 102-105, 2003.
5. Sun, LH. New challenge for Obamacare: enrollees who don't understand their insurance plans. *Washington Post*, July 16, 2014.
6. Weinberg, SK. The SCOTUS Hobby Lobby decision: A great opportunity to push for national public health coverage. *Health Care for All-Washington Newsletter,* Summer 2014.
7. Friedman, G. Funding HR 676: The Expanded and Improved Medicare for All Act. How We Can Afford a National Single-Payer Health Plan. Physicians for a National Health Plan. Chicago, Il, July 31, 2013. Available at: http: //www.pnhp. org/sites/default/files/Funding%20HR%20676-Friedman-final-7.31.13.pdf
8. `PNHP. The National Health Program Reader. Leadership Training Institute. Chicago, Il. Physicians for a National Health Program, November 5, 2010, with later updates.
9. Schiff, GD, Bindman, AB, Brennan, TA et al. A better quality alternative: single-payer national health system reform. *JAMA* 272 (10): 803-808, 1994.
10. Geyman, JP. *Breaking Point: How the Primary Care Crisis Endangers the Lives of Americans*. Friday Harbor, WA. Copernicus Healthcare, 2011.
11. Ibid # 5.
12. Dr. Gerald Friedman, personal communication, January 26, 2014.
13. Dickman, SL, Himmelstein, DU, McCormick, D et al. Health and financial harms of 25 states' decision to opt out of Medicaid. *Health Affairs Blog*, January 30, 2014.
14. Schiff, G. Medical malpractice: health care quality and reform. *Forum Report # 4*, Physicians for a National Health Program, New York Metro, 2003.
15. Canadian Health Services Research Foundation. *Mythbusters:* Medical malpractice suits plague Canada, 2006.
16. Adelman, SH, Westerlund, L. The Swedish Patient Compensation System: A viable alternative to the U.S. tort system. *Bull Am Coll Surg* 89 (1): 25-30, 2004.
17. Rowan, K, McAlpine, DD, Blewett, LA. Access and cost barriers to mental health care, by insurance status, 1999 to 2010. *Health Affairs* 32 (10): 1723-1730, 2013.
18. Geyman, JP. *Do Not Resuscitate: Why the Health Insurance Industry Is Dying and How We Must Replace It.* Monroe, ME. Common Courage Press, 2008, p. 187.

19. Loten, A. Kicked off group health plans, some owners face a tough choice. *Wall Street Journal*, August 7, 2014: B1.

20. Reuther, W., as cited by Gladwell, M. The risk pool: What's behind Ireland's economic miracle and the GM's financial crisis? *The New Yorker*, August 28, 2006, p. 35.

21. Woolhandler, S, Himmelstein, DU. Administrative work consumes one-sixth of U.S. physicians' working hours and lowers their career satisfaction. *Intl J Health Services* 44 (4), 2014.

22. Blendon, RJ, Benson, JM, Hero, JO. Public trust in physicians—U.S. medicine in international perspective. *N Engl J Med,* October 23, 2014.

Chapter 15

POLITICAL PROSPECTS
FOR NATIONAL HEALTH INSURANCE

The main issue that I have is that in America today the middle class is disappearing while the gap between rich and poor is growing wider. We need more people in politics working for ordinary people and not just the top 1 percent. . . . I believe that all over this country—in so-called Red States and in so-called Blue States—people are profoundly disgusted about what is happening and that they want real change.[1]

—Sen. Bernie Sanders (Ind. Vermont)

One positive aspect of the current chaos is that it is generating dissatisfaction on all sides. Sooner rather than later we are going to have to develop a national health plan. The design and implementation of such a plan will be an exciting task of the fairly near future, I believe. This country has tremendous wisdom and tremendous goodness. Eventually they will triumph in health care.[2]

—Dr. Avedis Donabedian, former professor emeritus
at the University of Michigan School of Public Health
and widely regarded as the father of quality assurance
in U.S.health care.

The above quote by an international expert in quality assessment of health care was made during an interview just a month before his death in November 2000 from prostate cancer. He was very knowledgable of the strengths and problems of different health care systems and an advocate for social justice in health care. His words of 15 years ago could not be more relevant today. We certainly have enough chaos to go around, and need to find our way out of it, the sooner the better.

The goals of this chapter are four-fold: (1) to briefly describe the political landscape in the aftermath of the 2014 mid-term elections; (2) to consider the corrupting influence of money in politics following the Citizens United and McCutcheon rulings of the U.S. Supreme Court; (3) to discuss the forces for and against NHI; and (4) to outline some of the next steps that can lead to real health care reform in this country.

THE NEW POLITICAL LANDSCAPE

The ACA was a central issue in a political crossfire even before the start of the 2014 midterm election cycle. Republicans at first wanted to repeal the legislation altogether, with the Republican-controlled House voting more than 50 times to repeal it. But many Republicans backed off repeal efforts after the first open enrollment period successfully enrolled 8 million Americans and after Medicaid actually expanded in many states. Then the House passed a resolution to sue President Obama over his failing to enforce the employer mandate of the ACA, claiming that his administration's changes in 2013 "created his own law" without Congressional action.[3] Meanwhile and predictably, the Republican attack on the ACA included charges that it is a government takeover, socialized medicine, too expensive, and too complicated. Hypocritically, Republicans also rail against proposed cuts to Medicare Advantage overpayments under the ACA.

Never mind that the ACA is essentially a conservative bill originally brought forward by the Heritage Foundation years ago as a way to keep private insurers alive and avoid single-payer national health insurance. Paul Krugman has pointed out the logic of the ACA as well as the Massachusetts 2006 Romney plan as the conservative alternative:

ObamaRomneyCare is a three-legged stool that needs all three legs. If you want to cover preexisting conditions, you must have the mandate; if you want the mandate, you must have subsidies. If you think there's some magic market-based solution that obviates the stuff conservatives don't

like while preserving the stuff they like, you're deluding
yourself. . . . What this means in practice is that any notion
the Republicans will go beyond trying to sabotage the law
and come up with an alternative is fantasy.[4]

In fact, Republicans have still not come up with an alternative to the ACA. Their warmed-over proposals—that have never
worked for many years—include further privatization of Medicare and Medicaid, increased cost-sharing with patients having
more "skin in the game", health savings accounts, vouchers for
Medicare, and depending on free health care markets to rein in
costs through "competition." Representative Paul Ryan (R-WI),
House Budget Committee chairman and an aspiring presidential
contender in 2016, took center stage with his austerity budget
that would cut $5 trillion in spending over the next ten years. The
Ryan budget would repeal the ACA and convert Medicare into
a premium support system in which seniors 65 and older would
buy private insurance with federal subsidies. Traditional Medicare would be weakened and premiums would increase, as would
seniors' out-of-pocket costs. The Ryan budget would also require
steep cuts in Medicaid, extend block grants to states, and cut funding for food stamps.[5,6]

The Ryan budget, of course, gave Democrats many ways to
counter-attack. They courted the senior vote by fighting against
Ryan's voucher plan for Medicare, defended the ACA and Medicaid expansion, supported an increase in the minimum wage, and
fought against cuts in food stamps. Democrats in southern states
running for re-election were on a hot seat over the ACA. They had
to be careful how much they supported the ACA, with some join-
ing the Republicans' fight against the ACA's cuts in Medicare Advantage overpayments.[7] At the same time, there were some brave
Democrats, such as Senator Mark Pryor (D-ARK), who came out
in support of raising the minimum wage and against privatizing
Medicare.

Although Obamacare was initially predicted by many to be a
central issue in the 2014 mid-term election cycle, it faded as public polling showed mixed results and as other issues came to the

fore, such as the wars and Ebola. The political benefits that Democrats hoped the ACA would bring failed to materialize as multiple polls taken between 2010 and a month before the election showed increasing opposition to the ACA.[8] Many Democrats were wary of defending it as Republicans continued their attacks against it. On the other side, the ACA was losing its campaign punch for Republicans, as they were forced to recognize that many people were benefitting from it.[9]

As we know too well, the Republicans swept the midterms, gaining a solid majority in the Senate and expanding their majority in the House. At the same time, they gained governorships in such influential states as Illinois and Massachusetts, while adding to the list of potential presidential candidates for 2016. Republicans now head state governments in two-thirds of the nation's states, and both houses of 30 state legislatures are controlled by Republicans.

Exit interviews from the midterms revealed a sharply divided electorate on most key issues. Concerning the ACA, most polls showed either non-support or that the law "didn't go far enough." Beyond the congressional races, there were some interesting results on some state ballot measures related to health care, but with no clear theme on the political spectrum. As examples, North Dakota and Colorado rejected so-called "personhood" amendments that would have amended their state constitutions to recognize rights for unborn fetuses.[10]

Voter turnout for the 2014 midterms was the lowest since the 1940s, especially among young voters. Voters under age 30 made up just 12 percent of all those who voted, compared to people age 60 and older accounting for almost 40 percent of total voters. Young voters were turned off by candidates' failure to address fundamental issues of the day, such as growing inequality, the student debt crisis, and underemployment. Carl Gibson, age 26, co-founder of U.S. Uncut, a nationwide creative direct-action movement, issued this challenge to Democrats:

We just didn't vote for Democrats who haven't done anything for us since we voted for them in 2012, and who brazenly took our votes for granted this year . . . You Democrats looked pitiful in the year leading up to the midterms. You didn't seem to stand for anything in particular, you just pointed the finger at the other guy, told us they were bad, and that you weren't like them. That's not enough. Take a risk, be bold.[11]

What can we expect of the new political landscape? That is the still unanswerable question raising speculation in all quarters. Now the Republicans have to govern, and the battle lines are drawn between the White House and Congress. The 2016 campaigns are already underway. Compromises over "common ground" will cut both ways, and the Republicans do not want to give Obama credit for anything in the final two years of his presidency. Democrats can filibuster objectionable bills in the Senate and President Obama can veto any bills that overcome the filibuster. Republicans can attach "poison pill" riders to must-pass legislation through the reconciliation process, and potentially force the president to sign them into law because of the necessity of the major legislation, such as a must-pass budget. Given all these complicated maneuvers, with increasing stakes amidst 2016 election campaigns, we are likely to see ongoing political gridlock.

Concerning the ACA, Jonathan Cohn of the *New Republic* gives us this insightful forecast of what Republicans will try to do, based on his conversations with health care experts and lobbyists:

- Repeal the individual mandate.
- Repeal or modify the employer mandate (e.g. change the threshold to a 40 hour week)
- Eliminate "risk corridors."
- Repeal the medical device tax.
- Abolish the Independent Payment Advisory Board (IPAB)
- Introduce a "copper plan" with 50 percent actuarial value.[12]

It now appears that the ACA will not be repealed altogether, but that some of the above changes, if adopted, may diminish its impact. Private insurers are eyeing new markets during the second enrollment period, while hospitals are seeing increased revenues with the expansion of Medicaid. A post-election consensus of Wall Street and business leaders finds little appetite for wholesale changes in the ACA.[13] In fact, the private health insurance industry and its shareholders see ongoing billions of new revenues from expanded markets. Wall Street is exuberant about the prospects for the industry with the Republicans gaining control of both houses of Congress. Within 24 hours of Senator Mitch McConnell being confirmed as the incoming Senate Majority Leader, share prices of five of the six largest for-profit insurers reached their highest points in a year, As one indication of the new (subsidized) bonanza for the industry, UnitedHealth stock went up by 315 percent since the ACA was enacted in 2010.[14]

What may become a bigger problem for the ACA could happen, however, when the U.S. Supreme Court hears a Republican-backed appeal that would block people in 36 states from getting tax subsidies to help them afford health insurance through the exchanges. A ruling on that question could destabilize insurance markets across the country, leading to higher insurance premiums and more uncompensated care for hospitals.[15]

Looking ahead to the 2016 election cycle, we see a number of Republican presidential candidates warming up in the bullpen, all well to the right on the political spectrum. Potential candidates range from Senator Ted Cruz to Representative Paul Ryan, and Governors Rick Scott, Scott Walker, and Chris Christie, to former Governor Jeb Bush. Among Democrats, Hillary Clinton seems inevitable, though many hope that Sen. Elizabeth Warren and Independent Sen. Bernie Sanders will run in order to put forward a more progressive agenda for the country.

Two recent articles bring us a broad historical perspective of American politics that is relevant today in looking at the prospects of the health care issue and other major issues of our time. Robert Kuttner wonders why the central economic fact of the last 40 years in this country—stagnation and decline of earnings of the working and middle class—has not become the leading issue in today's politics. He answers this question in two ways: (1) a prevailing view among the public, encouraged by Republicans, that the government should and cannot play much of a part in the economy; and (2) that persistent divisions of race, including a nativist backlash against immigrants, undermine "a common politics of uplift for working Americans generally." As Republicans press home their attack on "big government," he notes that the Obama administration's economic policies have been "reduced mostly to a politics of gesture." Kuttner further observes:

Reform eras are always a dance of social movements and inspired presidents. Movements can push for frame-breaking ideas, but only a president can make them mainstream, , , , [Obama's presidency] turned out to be too weak a politics or a set of policies for a crisis that required more.[16]

Paul Starr gives us an overview that sees the political gravity today as well right of center, despite demographic changes that favor Democrats. He notes that, since 2006, Democrats have an 18-point advantage among young adults overall, while seniors have become more Republican. In his words:

Routinely, Republicans criticize Obama and the Democrats for failing to cut Medicare and Social Security and the next day run TV ads warning seniors that Obama and the Democrats are cutting Medicare and Social Security. That gambit may work when Republicans are out of power, but if they have to govern, they will need to choose between the ideological and demographic parts of their base.[17]

THE CORRUPTING INFLUENCE OF MONEY IN POLITICS

The 2014 midterm elections were the most expensive midterms in U.S. history, driven especially by the growth of outside spending and Dark Money, for a total cost of $4 billion. More than a third of that money was channeled through Dark Money groups, without disclosure of their donors, targeting a small number of closely contested races.[18]

As is now only too obvious, our democracy is now doubly challenged by two actions of the U.S. Supreme Court, both 5-4—the 2010 Citizens United v. FEC ruling that allows corporations, unions and issue advocacy organizations to spend unlimited amounts of money to influence political campaigns, followed by the April 2014 McCutcheon v. FEC ruling that permits a small number of billionaires and millionaires to pump even more money into political campaigns. The super-wealthy can now donate $3.6 million directly to candidates and parties in a single election cycle, and because of Citizens United, much more to "independent" groups like Super PACs.[19] The McCutcheon ruling threw out the previous $123,200 cap on individual giving in an election cycle as a violation of free speech.[20] Writing for the majority, Chief Justice John Roberts said: "the government may not seek to limit the appearance of mere influence or access."[21] Bill Moyers was quick to point out the obvious result of this ruling: "You're entitled to all the free speech you can buy."[22]

As Robert Reich wrote in reaction to these rulings:

> *In turn-of-the-century America, when the lackeys of robber barons literally placed sacks of cash on the desks of pliant legislators, the great jurist Louis Brandeis warned that the nation faced a choice. 'We may have democracy, or we may have wealth concentrated in the hands of a few, but we can't have both'". . . In the short term, McCutcheon v. FEC might make it easier for today's robber barons to take over American politics. But by inviting them to corrupt our democracy so brazenly, it also might fuel a popular backlash leading to a new era of reform. It has happened before.*[23]

The rapidly widening income gap in the U.S. population adds fuel to this political fire. Figure 15.1 shows the incomes of the wealthiest 0.01 percent as multiples of average incomes from 1920 to 2012, based on the work of Thomas Piketty, professor at the Paris School of Economics and author of the widely acclaimed classic book, *Capital in the Twenty-First Century*. As Paul Krugman warns in his *New York Review of Books* review of the book:

FIGURE 15.1

Income of the Wealthiest 0.01% as Multiple of Average Income, 1920-2012

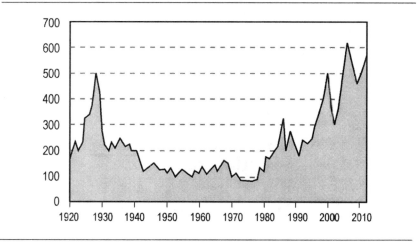

Source: Piketty, T, Saez, E. Available at
htpp://elsa.berkeley.edu/~saez/tabfig2005prel.xls

The big idea of [this book] is that we haven't just gone back to the nineteenth-century levels of income inequality, we're also on a path back to 'patrimonial capitalism', in which the commanding heights of the economy are controlled not by talented individuals but by family dynasties. . . The current generation of the very rich in America may consist largely of executives rather than rentiers, people who live off accumulated capital, but these executives have heirs. And America two decades from now could be a rentier-dominated society even more unequal than Belle Epoque Europe.[24]

Since the financial meltdown in 2008, we have seen a reverse transfer from the poor and middle class to the very rich. Today, America's richest 1 percent have made more than the cost of all U.S. social programs, including Social Security, Medicare, Medicaid and our entire safety net, with almost none of their great wealth going to innovation or jobs.[25]

As we know too well, the claim by conservatives for the last four decades is that income inequality doesn't matter that much, that the wealthy are necessary to create jobs and lift the economy. However, if we look at the top tax rates and GDP growth over the last 100 years (Figure 15.2), we can see that low taxes on the wealthy do not bring economic growth. The old, by now discredited "trickle down" theory should be put to rest.

FIGURE 15.2

Highest Marginal Tax Rate
Vs. Average Per Capita GDP Growth
1913-2013

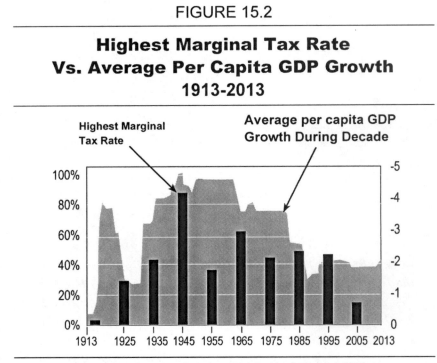

Source: Adapted from Tax Policy Center and Left Business Observer, 2011.

So yes, we have already lost much of our cherished democracy. Multi-national corporations outsource our jobs, reduce work force and wages in this country, and shift large amounts of revenue to off-shore tax havens while paying minimal taxes here. They lobby for more corporate tax breaks and game whatever tax loopholes they can. A good example is General Electric, which declared profits of more than $27 billion over the past five years, yet paid nothing in taxes and received more than $3 billion in tax refunds.[26] Meanwhile, our big corporations, including Koch Industries, reap millions from the ACA, even as they appropriate large sums to Republican candidates committed to repealing the law.[27]

As a result of all this, the ordinary voter has little if any influence on policy issues, dominated as politics are by a small number of wealthy elites. A recent study by two researchers—Martin Gilens of Princeton University and Benjamin Page of Northwestern University, concludes that:

> *Majorities of the American public actually have little influence over the policies our government adopts. Americans do enjoy many features central to democratic governance, such as regular elections, freedom of speech and association, and a widespread (if still contested) franchise. But we believe that if policymaking is dominated by powerful business organizations and a small number of affluent Americans, then America's claims to being a democratic society are seriously threatened.[28]*

FORCES FOR AND AGAINST NHI
On the support side.

Americans have shown high levels of support for a national health insurance program since the 1940s, when 74 percent of the public supported a proposal for NHI.[29] Since then, a majority of the public has supported NHI in one after another national poll. Table 15.1 shows these results from 1980 to 2000.[30,31] As an interesting comparison, Medicare was supported by 61 percent of respondents when it was enacted in 1965.[32] In 2006, when asked "Would you prefer the current health insurance system or a universal coverage program like Medicare that is government-run and financed by taxpayers?", 56 percent of respondents supported NHI.[33] A 2009 CBS News/*New York Times* poll found that the proportion of respondents favoring NHI increased from 40 percent in 1979 to 59 percent in 2009.[34] Still more recently, a 2013 CNN/ORC poll found that many who oppose the ACA support NHI. (Figure 15.3)[35]

TABLE 15.1

American's Attitudes About National Health Insurance, 1980-2000

National Health Insurance, financed by tax money, and paying for most forms of health care[a]

	Favor	Oppose	No Opinion
1980 (February)	50%	41%	9%
1980 (March)	46%	43%	11%
1981	52%	37%	11%
1990 (March-April)	56%	34%	10%
1990 (October)	64%	27%	8%
1991 (June)	60%	30%	10%
1991 (August)	54%	33%	12%
1992 (January)	65%	26%	9%
1992 (July)	66%	25%	9%
1993 (January)	63%	26%	11%
1993 (March)	59%	29%	12%
1995	53%	39%	8%
2000 (August)			
General public	56%	32%	12%
Registered voters	54%	34%	12%

Sources: Blendon, R. J., & Benson, J. M. (2001). Americans' views on health policy: A fifty-year historical perspective. *Health Affairs (Millwood)*, 20(2), 35. Reprinted with permission.
CBS News/*New York Times* polls (1980-95); Harvard School of Public Health/ ICR poll (2000).

FIGURE 15.3

Many Who Oppose Obamacare Prefer Single-Payer

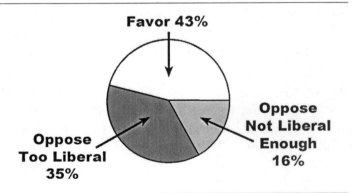

Favor 43%

Oppose Not Liberal Enough 16%

Oppose Too Liberal 35%

Source: *New York Times*, based on CNN/ORC poll, May 17-18, 2013.

A majority of physicians and other health professionals support NHI. They provide all of our health care and are increasingly fed up with their daily hassles with the expanding bureaucracy of our complex and dysfunctional multi-payer financing system. Activist positions for single-payer NHI have been taken by a growing number of professional organizations, including the American College of Physicians (ACP), the second largest physician organization in the country with 137,000 members, Physicians for a National Health Program (PNHP) with 19,000 members, the American Public Health Association (APHA), the American Psychiatric Association (APA), the American Society of Clinical Oncology (ASCO), and the California Nurses Association (CNA). A 2008 study of more than 2,200 U.S. physicians in 13 specialties found that 59 percent support NHI.[36]

A growing number of medical leaders are taking strong leadership positions in calling for single-payer NHI, as these quotes illustrate:

With the costs of cancer care skyrocketing out of control, most people with cancer are burdened not only physically but also financially. They delay or do not receive care due to their inability to pay. . . . The situation is worsening. We need a fundamental shift in our approach to funding health care in the United States.[37]

—Ray Drasga, M.D, long-time community oncologist
and co- author of an article in the Journal of
Oncology Practice calling for his specialty society
(ASCO) to endorse a single-payer system.

[Answering the question "what is the biggest barrier to your practicing medicine today?"]: The lack of a single-payer system. We waste enormous amounts of time and energy dealing with insurance companies, whose major goal is figuring out how not to cover patients.[38]

—Steven Nissen, M.D., chairman of the Department of
Cardiovascular Medicine at the Cleveland Clinic and past
president of the American College of Cardiology

[Answering the same question put to Dr. Nissen above]: Without a doubt, it is lack of access for many patients, especially the un- and underinsured.[39]

—Eric Matteson, M.D., chair of rheumatology and
professor of medicine at the Mayo Clinic

Physicians should be in charge of health care and not the insurance companies and hospital systems. . . .I would submit to you that it is un-American to allow many of our citizens to be uninsured, to shunt money away from a strong military in order to support a bloated, inefficient and fraud-laden health care system, not to be open and above board with the cost of what we do, the expense of that service and the profit that we make. Mostly, it is un-American to let this outrageous health care injustice continue.[40]

—David May, M.D., Ph.D., practicing cardiologist, a
Republican, and chair of the Board of Governors of the
American College of Cardiologists

The 30-page H.R. 676, the single payer bill of Rep. John Conyers Jr., a Michigan Democrat, shows how simple it is to cover everyone. It provides savings through quality care—including protection from harmful overuse and efficient, timely management of chronic disease—as well as savings through national monopsony buying power and freedom from insurance business profits.[41]

—James Burdick, M.D., Professor of Surgery, Johns
Hopkins University School of Medicine

[Responding to a question about the start of health insurance under the ACA): I think there should be a single-payer system. And, increasingly you're seeing physicians in their late 50s, 60s, and 70s who are saying, 'You know what, we got it wrong; we should have taken Medicare, expanded it, and done it smarter.[42]

—Dr. Nancy Snyderman, NBC's chief medical editor

And there are many other opinion leaders in other walks of life who have come out in strong support of single-payer, including Colin Powell, who recently said:

I have benefitted from that kind of universal health care in my 55 years of public life. And I don't see why we can't do what Europe is doing, what Canada is doing, what South Korea is doing, what all these other places are doing.[43]

Some CEOs of large corporations have also seen single-payer to their advantage, such as Jack Smith, CEO of General Motors from 1992 to 2000, who said in the early 1990s: "I personally favor single payer." He understood only too well what his counterpart CEOs of GM, Ford and DaimlerChrysler in Canada knew— that single payer was a "strategic advantage for Canada."[44]

We are now seeing some hard-core conservatives coming out, even including Charles Krauthammer, *Washington Post* commentator, Fox News analyst, and a physician, who recently said:

Obamacare is such a clumsy beast that it will simply expire . . . and then the country's going to have a true choice between a single-payer system . . . [and] a free-market system.[45] *A single-payer system would at least have been logical and simple.*[46]

Another Republican, Geraldo Rivera, who has the show *Geraldo-at-Large* on Fox News Channel, has said:

I want everyone to have health care. I want single payer. I want Medicare for everybody. . . . This program (Obamacare) is deeply flawed, and I think part of the problem is we let the insurance industry write the legislation, and when the insurance industry writes the legislation, they stack the deck so they're the beneficiaries.[47]

Single payer NHI has the support of many organizations across our society, including Healthcare NOW!, Labor Campaign for Single-Payer Health Care, One Payer States, National Nurses

United, Physicians for a National Health Program, Progressive Democrats for America, and many others.

Forces Opposing NHI.

Given the above forces in support of NHI, we might ask why we didn't come to this solution long ago? The answer, of course, is the political power and money of corporate stakeholders who want to perpetuate the profits and waste of our market-based system as long as possible. The insurance industry, despite its protests about some details in the bill, is first in line among corporate stakeholders wanting to preserve the ACA against any possibility of the single-payer alternative.

Beyond the power and influence of money and lobbyists over the last three decades, a concerted system of messaging has kept progressive issues off the table. A recent Op-Ed by Dave Johnson of Campaign for America's Future gives us an insightful view of long-term opposition to single-payer, as well as other more progressive policy changes:

> *The Koch brothers, other billionaires and corporate groups have been remarkably successful in pushing Congress to pass legislation that helps their interests while hurting the rest of us. . . . [They] put their money into think tanks, communication outlets, publishers, various media, etc. with a long-term plan to change the way people see things. This 'apparatus' has pounded out corporate/conservative propaganda 24/7 for decades.*[48]

There are more than 20 right-wing think tanks that employ full-time health policy "scholars" to oppose NHI and advocate for privatization of health care, deregulation, and other market-based initiatives. These include the American Enterprise Institute, the Cato Institute, the Galen Institute, the Heartland Institute, the Heritage Foundation, the Manhattan Institute, the National Center for Policy Analysis, the Pacific Research Institute, the National Center for Public Policy Research, and Freedom Works Foundation (founded by Charles Koch). At the state level, the American

Legislative Exchange Council (ALEC), a spinoff of the Heritage Foundation, opposes single-payer initiatives and lobbies in support of private health insurance. Some, such as the Fraser Institute, the Discovery Institute, and Americans for Prosperity, disseminate disinformation concerning the Canadian single-payer system.[49]

This concerted effort by the right over the last three decades has won the day over liberals and progressives seeking a more progressive agenda. Dave Johnson further observes:

On [the left}, money, resources and effort tend to go into candidates, with so many people looking for a 'messiah' candidate to lead them out of the wilderness and somehow convince the public of the rightness of our cause. Then after the campaigns are over, the infrastructure dissolves, the expertise disperses, needing to be rebuilt from scratch two or four years later. It is a remarkably ineffective approach.[50]

THE ROAD AHEAD TO REAL
HEALTH CARE REFORM

In the aftermath of the 2014 mid-term elections, confusion and polarization reign over the fate of the Affordable Care Act. Some legislators and policymakers would still like to let the ACA run its course, betting that its benefits will exceed its limits over the long haul. Although Republicans may put forward another symbolic bill to repeal the ACA (knowing that it cannot pass into law), they will try to kill it by a thousand cuts if they can. But Republicans still have no credible plan to replace it. And as is made clear in earlier chapters, the ACA is too flawed, bureaucratic, wasteful, and expensive to either succeed for our population or be sustainable.

As this book goes to press, the U.S. Supreme Court is planning to hear a case, *King vs. Burwell,* which has to do whether or not tax credits apply only in the consumer marketplaces in the 16 states with their own exchanges, or can be available to consumers purchasing coverage on the 36 federal exchanges. The question turns on interpretation of these few words—[subsidies are available only in] "exchanges established by a state." A ruling is expected near the end of the Court's present term, in late June or early July of 2015.[51,52] This is a fundamental question for afford-ability of coverage under the ACA, and could cripple the law if the Justices rule that tax credits are only available through the state exchanges. In view of the Court's 5-4 ruling allowing states not to expand Medicaid, another such ruling against the ACA could be a crippling blow to the ACA.

Dr. Don McCanne, health policy expert and senior health policy fellow at PNHP, sums up the need to go beyond the ACA in this helpful way:

What successes are the ACA supporters touting?
- *Coverage of only about half of the uninsured*
- *Shift to underinsurance products*
- *Guaranteed issue of these underinsurance products*
- *Deductibles that keep patients away from care by erecting financial barriers*
- *Insurance subsidies that are inadequate*
- *Ultra-narrow networks that take away choice*
- *Insurance marketplaces that increase administrative com-plexity and waste*
- *Inadequate cost-containment policies (except for perverse higher deductibles)*

What are we not getting from ACA that we would be getting from single payer?
- *Truly universal coverage*
- *Dramatic reduction in administrative waste*
- *Removal of financial barriers to care*
- *Coverage of all essential health care services*
- *Free choice of hospitals and health care professionals*
- *Removal of the interventions and excesses of the private insurers*
- *Taxpayer financing based on ability to pay*
- *Infrastructure reform that would slow spending to sustain able levels[53]*

Financing reform through single-payer NHI is the key that will enable other essential reforms, including cost containment, shifting to a not-for-profit, evidence-based and service-oriented system, improving quality and outcomes of care, simplifying administration, and reducing health care bureaucracy. It will change how physicians are paid and establish global budgets for hospitals and other facilities. As this book goes to press, there are two bills pending in the U.S. Congress—the Improved and Expanded Medicare for All Act in the House (H.R. 676) and the American Health Security Act (S.1782) in the Senate.

Recent years have shown continued political gridlock in Washington, D.C. with both parties skirting the most important issues of our time—renewing the American dream for much of our population, campaign finance reform, breaking the vice-grip of corporate power, and restoring a vibrant democracy.

The health care debate is not a left vs. right issue, but a top-down one. As Howard Zinn reminded us, it is the ultimate measure of a democracy—"Democracy is not what governments do. It's what people do."[54]

Health care reform of the magnitude needed has failed for a century in this country, regardless of which party was in power, in each instance because of the lack of a strong social movement from below. Tommy Douglas, the pioneering leader in Canada who led the way to its national system of universal coverage, used this abbreviated political fable frequently during his long campaign for its passage:

Mouseland was a place where all the little mice lived and played, were born and died. And they lived much the same as you and I do. They had a Parliament and elections. They always elected a government made up of cats. The cats were nice fellows, but made good laws for cats, not mice. One law required for mouse holes to be big enough for a cat to get its paws into. Since round holes were bad, they tried square mouse holes, but they were twice as big as the round ones, and were even tougher on mice. Then they tried electing black cats, white cats, or coalitions of both. But the results were always the same until one of the mice had a better idea—elect mice instead of cats! But he was called a Bolshevik and jailed.

Tommy Douglas then ended this story with: "But I want to remind you, you can lock up a mouse or a man but you can't lock up an idea."[55]

A broad social movement can, and should, come out of several converging societal challenges, including reducing the widening income and opportunity gap that splits our society, the need for repeal of Citizens United and McCutcheon rulings by the U.S. Supreme Court, recognition of health care as a universal human need and right, raising the minimum wage, ending of corporate welfare, campaign finance reform, and creating jobs in the public sector, especially to rebuild the nation's eroding infrastructure. Opponents of the Occupy movement will tell us that that a broad social movement is impossible, since the Occupy effort sputtered out. But there is evidence to the contrary in our own history. Social Security, the New Deal, and civil rights legislation did not come out of nowhere. They were a democratic response to major national problems. Jim Hightower, bestselling author, radio commentator, syndicated columnist, and editor of the *Hightower Lowdown*, calls for a new wave of populism in these graphic words:

> *Populism is the un-corporate America. It is a distinctive, very progressive and very American democratic–ism that not only acts politically but also economically, socially and culturally. As old as the USA itself, populism has a rich egalitarian philosophy, a deep history, noble accomplishments, and a broad reach that cuts right through the conventional political boxes that are deliberately designed to divide us. . . . The recent rise of populist fervor is showing once again that the true political spectrum in our country is not right to left [but] from top to bottom. . . We need not fear talking to the people about even our strongest progressive proposals, for they're already with us—or ahead of us. Citizens United? Eighty percent want it repealed, including 76 percent of Republicans. Hike the minimum wage? Hell, yes—again including a majority of*

> *Republicans and even 42 percent of Tea Partiers. . . So*
> *we don't have to generate public support for a populist*
> *politics, for it's already in the hearts, minds and guts of*
> *the majority, though most don't know the name for it. . .*
> *Building a people's movement requires taking the long view.*
> *As my friend Willie Nelson has observed: "The early bird*
> *may get the worm, but the second mouse gets the cheese."*[56]

As Robert Reich looks at our present predicament, five years into our "recovery" that has decimated the middle class and further enriched the very rich, he notes the growth of a populist movement that is shifting from Democrat vs. Republican to populist vs. establishment—"those who think the game is rigged vs. those who do the rigging."[57]

Returning to health care, can we have any optimism that NHI can become a reality in the U.S., given the power and political track record of corporate interests over the last three decades? A resounding Yes!—for these reasons:

- The shortfalls and inevitable failure of the ACA to meet the public's needs at an affordable price will lead to a stark choice—in both major political parties—between single-payer and deregulated markets that are already discredited. This will give the Republican party a chance to live up to its credo of wanting efficiency, choice, affordability, value, fiscal responsibility, equity and accountability.
- Changing demographics will bring increased voting strength to many millions of working and middle-class Americans, especially including minorities and young people.
- With single-payer financing reform, we already have the building blocks for an excellent, more fair and humane health care system, including many fine hospitals with open beds, enough well-trained health professionals (except in primary care), and world-class research.
- We already have more than enough money in the system to achieve universal access to necessary care for all Americans and still reduce the deficit, as shown in Chapter 12.
- The potential of social media, especially twitter, is not yet

realized, and could be instrumental in building a broad-based social movement for change.

As they say, all politics are local, and we are seeing a remarkable and growing backlash to the corrupting power of money in politics. One recent example is the election of Tom Butt as the new mayor of Richmond, CA despite the multi-million dollar effort by Chevron Corp. to pack the City Council with compliant members.[58] As another example, sixteen states and more than 500 communities from the city of Los Angeles to the town of Mount Desert, Maine are calling for a constitutional amendment to restore the ability of cities, states and the federal government to regulate money in politics.[59] Still another example is in North Dakota, where Walmart spent about $7 million trying to overturn a 1963 law preventing chain pharmacies from operating in the state, a threat to independent pharmacies in the state. In a November 2014 referendum, North Dakota voters upheld the law, reassuring many local and rural pharmacists.[60]

Medicine can, and should, play an important role in leading toward improved access, quality and equity of health care for all Americans. So far most medical organizations have not taken up a leadership role to that end, still not seeing beyond their own self-interest. The late Dr. Arnold Relman, internist and former editor of *The New England Journal of Medicine*, who coined the term "medical-industrial complex" in 1980, leaves U.S. physicians with this challenge:

> *Physicians have a unique power to reshape the medical care system. They are what makes it work and are best qualified to use and evaluate its resources. But if they never unite to press for major reform, the future of health care in the United States will indeed be bleak. We will end up either with a system controlled by blind market forces or with a system entangled in complicated and intrusive government regulations. In either case it would be impossible to practice good patient-centered medicine, and the quality and effectiveness of our health care system would sink even lower among the ranks of developed countries. It is up to the medical profession to see that this does not happen.[61]*

We are on the verge of major political change. Figure 15.4 illustrates forces for and against health care reform. We need a major shift of the pendulum back to the needs of most Americans. These words by Lawrence Lessig, whom we met in earlier chapters, are right on target:

We need a politics that is not about politicians. We need a people who devote themselves to saving this republic without others wondering whether they are simply trying to secure a job for themselves. We need a way to engage that is not about just listening. We need to take responsibility for the government we ask the politicians to run. We need to fix it, and then give it back to them to run.
We citizens. You. Me. Us. [62]

And what kind of government should we demand through our active grassroots politics? These two observations more than two hundred years apart give us wise guidance:

Government is instituted for the common good; for the protection, safety, prosperity and happiness of the people; and not for the profit, honor, or private interest of any one man, family, or class of men." [63]

—John Adams, second president of the United States
(1797-1801) and one of our founding fathers

[In response to a question by Bill Moyers concerning the one question we should be thinking about in the aftermath of the financial meltdown of 2008-2009], James K. Galbraith, leading economist of our time, has this to say:

Where do we want to be in thirty years time? It's not a question of how we return to full employment prosperity in five years, but how we solve the fundamental problems that we face in a way that gives us a generation of steady progress, and living standards that people can accept, that they'll be happy with, while at the same time achieving sustainability and reestablishing the American position as a leading and responsible country in the world. . . . It's a test for the country as a whole, as to whether we have the capacity to state and pursue a truly public purpose. We've come through a generation where we have really denied the existence of a common good or a public purpose. And I think we've recognized that that path leads to collapse, the collapse that we've seen. And that the way out is to somehow reestablish for ourselves this vision of what we really could be.[64]

FIGURE 15.4

The Political Teeter-Totter
Where Will the Forces Go?

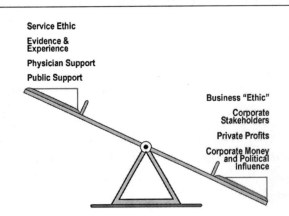

Service Ethic

Evidence & Experience

Physician Support

Public Support

Business "Ethic"

Corporate Stakeholders

Private Profits

Corporate Money and Political Influence

References

1. Queally, J. Bernie Sanders: I want to know if ordinary people are ready to stand and fight. *Common Dreams*, August 28, 2014.
2. Donabedian, A. As interviewed by Mullan, F. A founder of quality assessment encounters a troubled system firsthand. *Health Affairs* (Millwood) 20 (1): 131, 2001.
3. Dennis, S. House Resolution authorizes suing Obama over Affordable Care Act. *Roll Call*, July 10, 2014.
4. Krugman, P. Obamacare: The unknow ideal. http://krugman.blogs.nytimes.com/2014/03/31/obamacare-the-unknown-ideal/
5. Weisman, J. Ryan's budget would cut $5 trillion in spending over a decade. *New York Times*, April 1, 2014.
6. Medicare Watch. More of the same in House Republican budget proposal. *Medicare Rights Center*, April 3, 2014.
7. Peterson, K, Mathews, AW. Some Democrats fight Obama over Medicare. *Wall Street Journal*, April 7, 2014: A4.
8. Wheaton, S. Obamacare brings Democrats backlash, not benefits. *Politico*, October 29, 2014.
9. Memoli,. MA, Mascaro, L. Obamacare loses some of its campaign punch for Republicans. *Los Angeles Times*, August 3, 2014.

10. Rovner, J. Voters provide mixed messages on health ballot measures. *Kaiser Health News*, November 5, 2014.

11. Gibson, C. as quoted by Salzillo, L. 26-ear old founder of U.S. Uncut sends open letter to Democrats on young voter disillusion. *Daily Kos*, November 8, 2o14.

12. Cohn, J. This is how the new GOP Senate will try to dismantle Obamacare. *New Republic*, November 4, 2014.

13. Schwartz, ND, Krauss, C. Business leaders cautiously expect G.O.P. win to open some doors. *New York Times*, November 5, 2014.

14. Potter, W. Health insurers win midterm elections. *The Progressive Populist*, December 15, 2014, p. 10.

15. Stohr, G. Obamacare faces new threat as Supreme Court weighs appeal. *Bloomberg*, October 30, 2014.

16. Kuttner, R. The hidden history of prosperity. *The American Prospect*, May/June: 41-48, 2014.

17. Starr, P. Moving left to the center. *The American Prospect* May/June: 5, 2014.

18. Weisman, R. There is a way forward. *Public Citizen*, November 5, 2014.

19. Graves, L. Supreme Court continues to corrupt democracy with latest ruling. *Center for Media and Democracy*, April 2, 2014.

20. Bravin, J, Nelson, CM. High court ends limit on donations. *Wall Street Journal*, April 4, 2014: A1.

21. Scherer, M. Money talks: a divided Supreme Court loosens the reins on campaign cash—again. *Time*, April 14, 2014, p. 14.

22. Moyers, B. quote from billmoyers.com, April 6, 2014.

23. Reich, R. Selling democracy caused backlash once, might again. *San Francisco Chronicle*, April 13, 2014.

24. Krugman, P. Review of Capital in the Twenty-First Century by Thomas Piketty. *New York Review of Books*, May 8, 2014.

25. Buchheit, P. Infuriating facts about our disappearing middle-class wealth. *Nation of Change*, November 3, 2014.

26. Borosage, R. Corporate tax breaks: how Congress rigs the rules. *Nation of Change*, April 30, 2014.

27. Dispatches. Obamacare critics, including Kochs, accept subsidies. *The Progressive Populist* 20 (8): 5, May 1, 2014.

28. Gilens, M, Page, BI. Testing theories of American politics: elites, interest groups, and average citizens. *Perspectives on Politics*, Fall 2014.

29. Steinmo, S, Watts, J. It's the institutions, stupid! Why comprehensive national health insurance always fails in America. *J Health Politics*, Policy and Law 20: 329, 1995.

30. Blendon, RJ, Benson, JM. Americans' views on health policy: A fifty-year perspective. *Health Affairs* (Millwood) 20 (2): 35, 2001.

31. CBS News/New York Times polls (1980-1995); Harvard School of Public Health/ICR poll (2000).

32. Ibid # 28.

33. ABC News Poll/USA Today/*Kaiser Survey*, September, 2006.

34. CBS News/*New York Times* Poll, February 1, 2009.

35. New York Times, based on CNN/ORC poll, May 17-18, 2013.

36. Carroll, AE, Ackermann, RT. Support for national health insurance among U.S. physicians: five years later. *Ann Intern Med* 1481: 566-567, 2008.

37. Drasga, RE, Einhorn, LH. Why oncologists should support single-payer national health insurance. *J Oncol Pract*, January 17, 2014.

38. Neale, T. 10 Questions: Steven Nissen, M.D. *MedPage Today*, December 5, 2013.
39. Walsh, N. 10 Questions: Eric Matteson, M.D. *MedPage Today*, December 27, 2013.
40. May, D. I am a Republican ... can we talk about a single-payer system? ACC in Touch blog, *American College of Cardiology*, April 23, 2013.
41. Burdick, JF. Getting serious about a single payer system. *The Baltimore Sun*, May 1, 2014.
42. Snyderman, N. Review of the chief health stories of 2013, December 30, 2013. www.msnbc.com/morning-joe
43. Nader, R. Colin Powell, General Motors and single-payer, December 13, 2013. action@singlepayeraction.org
44. Ibid # 41.
45. Clyne, M. Krauthammer: Obama's plan is to semi-nationalize healthcare. *Newmax*, April 22, 2014.
46. Carruthers, W. Krauthammer: Obamacare; single-payer would've been 'logical, simple'. *Newsmax*, March 24, 2014.
47. Rivera, G. Geraldo Rivera, November 1, 2013.
48. Johnson, D. Let's stop searching for a 'messiah' and build a movement. *Nation of Change*, May 25, 2014.
49. Skala, N, Gray, C. Right-wing "think " tanks and health policy. *The National Health Program Reader*. Chicago, IL. Physicians for a National Health Program, 2010, pp. 472-474.
50. Ibid # 46.
51. Denniston, L. Court to rule on health care subsidies. SCOTUSblog, November 7, 2014.
52. Rovner, J. In surprise move, Supreme Court will examine key part of health law. *Kaiser Health News*, November 7, 2014.
53. McCanne, D. Comment on Quote-of-the-Day, July 25, 2014.
54. Zinn, H, as cited in Moyers, B. Howard Zinn interview. *Truthout*, December 14, 2009.
55. Lingenfelter, D. The Story of Mouseland. Saskatchewan New Democrats. Accessed at http://www.saskndp.com/history/mouseland.php3 on January 4, 2010; full copy of that fable is available from that source.
56. Hightower, J. Time for a Populist Revival!: This old American tradition already has broad, deep support at the grassroots. *The Nation*, March 24, 2014, pp. 12-17.
57. Reich, R. Six principles of the new populism. *The Progressive Populist*, June 15, 2014, p. 12.
58. Gonzales, R. Chevron Corp. spends big, and loses big, in a City Council race. NPR—The Two Way, November 5, 2014.
59. Nichols, N, McChesney, RW. Dollarocracy: The squabbling of Democrats and Republicans has become a sideshow to the theater of plutocracy. *The Nation*. September 30, 2013, pp. 22-25.
60. Hansen, M, Schultz, K. 6 ways Americans voted against corporate power in the most expensive midterm elections ever. *Common Dreams*, November 6, 2014.
61. Relman, A. Physicians and politics. JAMA Internal Medicine, June 2, 2014.
62. Lessig, L. Republic Lost: How Money Corrupts Congress—and a Plan to Stop It. New York. Twelve. *Hatchette Book Group*, 2011, pp. 316-317.
63. Adams, J. As quoted by Hartmann, T. A red privatization story. *The Progressive Populist*, November 15, 2014, p. 11.
64. Galbraith, JK. As quoted by Bill Moyers in Bill Moyers Journal: The Conversation Continues. New York. *The New Press*, 2011, p. 245.

GLOSSARY

Accountable care organization (ACO): These are loosely designed managed care organizations involving hospital systems, physicians, and insurers, established under the ACA in an effort to contain health care costs. They are expected to provide care for a population of at least 5,000 people for a period of at least three years, with the goal to improve coordination and quality of care in and out of the hospital.

Actuarial value: The percentage of total average health care costs that a health plan will pay for covered services. The ACA set up four "metal" levels of health plans through the exchanges—ranging from bronze, which covers only 60 percent of costs, to platinum, which covers 90 percent of costs.

Adverse selection: This occurs when lower-risk individuals are split off by insurers from a larger risk pool in order to minimize their financial risk and increase their profits. The smaller risk pool of higher-risk individuals that results requires higher costs of treatment. Adverse selection is the Achilles' heel of capitation, since for-profit HMOs and some physicians are often tempted to selectively care for healthier patients while avoiding the care of sicker patients.

America's Health Insurance Plans (AHIP): This is the insurance industry's national trade group representing about 1,300 private insurance companies. It was formed in 2003 by the merger of the American Association of Health Plans (AAHP) and the Health Insurance Association of America (HIAA).

Capitation: A method of payment for patient care services used by managed care organizations, such as health maintenance organizations (HMOs), to reimburse providers under contractual agreements. Payment rates are set in advance, and are paid monthly or annually regardless of what services are actually provided to covered patients.

Consumer Directed Health Care (CDHC): A strategy intended to contain health care costs by shifting more responsibility to consumers in choosing and paying for their own health care. This theory of cost-containment has been supported by many economists and most conservatives for years, but has failed as a cost-containment measure while leading many lower-income patients to delay or forego necessary care.

Co-insurance: This refers to the percentage of health care costs which are not covered by insurance and which the individual must pay. Many insurance plans cover 80 percent of the costs of hospital and physician care, leaving 20 percent to be paid by patients or by supplemental insurance.

Community rating: A method for setting premiums for health insurance based on the average cost of health care for the covered population in a geographic area. This method shares risk across all covered individuals, whether sick or well, so that the healthy help to subsidize care of the sick who otherwise may not be able to afford coverage on their own. Community rating was abandoned by most private health insurers after the 1960s, as experience rating spread throughout the industry.

Cost effectiveness: When applied to health care, cost-effectiveness attempts to estimate the value for expenditures on procedures or services that is returned to patients, such as longer life, better quality of life, or both. Cost-effectiveness analysis (CEA) is the scientific technique used to measure costs and efficacy of alternative treatments in order to estimate their economic value, which then are typically measured in quality-adjusted life years (QALYs).

Co-payment: Flat fee charged directly to patients whenever they seek health care services or drug prescriptions regardless of their insurance coverage. In today's environment, co-payments are increasing across the health care marketplace to the point of being a financial barrier to care for many lower-income people.

Cost-sharing: This refers to requirements that patients pay directly out-of-pocket for some portion of their health care costs. The level of cost-sharing varies considerably from one health plan to another, and for many people is another financial barrier to access to necessary health care.

Death spiral: This term describes the progressive effects of adverse selection in shrinking a risk pool into a smaller population of high-risk individuals requiring expensive care. As a result of "cherry picking" by for-profit health insurers, public programs such as traditional Medicare are placed at risk because of reduced cross subsidies from the healthy to the sick.

Deductible: Out-of-pocket costs which patients must pay before their insurance coverage kicks in for subsequent costs. This amount is required to be met each year. The trend today is toward plans with high deductibles, some even up to $5,000 or more, constituting yet another financial barrier to care.

Defined benefits: This term is applied when an insurance plan offers a pre-determined set of benefits to all enrollees. Traditional Medicare is such an example, with covered benefits authorized by law.

Defined contributions: This is the polar opposite from defined benefits. In this instance, a fixed set of benefits is not provided by the insurer, whether public or private. Instead a defined contribution is made toward the costs of coverage, such as by an employer or a privatized public plan. See also Premium Support and Vouchers.

The Emergency Medical Treatment and Active Labor Act (EMTALA): This was enacted by Congress in 1986 in order to ensure public access to emergency services regardless of ability to pay. Medicare-participating hospitals that offer emergency services are required to provide stabilizing treatment for all emergency medical conditions, including active labor.

Employer mandate: A policy that requires all or most employers to provide health insurance for their employees. The Affordable Care Act includes this approach, but allows some exceptions to this requirement, which has also been delayed for a year.

Employer sponsored insurance (ESI): A voluntary system established during the wartime economy of the 1940s whereby many employers have provided health insurance coverage to their employees. This system has been gradually unraveling for years, now covering less than two-thirds of the non-elderly workforce, with many employers covering less through defined contribution and high-deductible plans.

Employee Retirement Income Security Act of 1974 (ERISA): Enacted in 1974 before the advent of managed care, ERISA was originally intended to protect pension plans, but soon became a loophole in states' attempts to regulate abuses by private health insurers. Under ERISA, all self-funded health plans are exempt from state regulations, as are many managed care organizations. ERISA does not apply to Medicare, Medicaid, and insurance provided by government employers.

Experience rating: This is the current norm in private U.S. health insurance markets, as opposed to the community rating tradition originally established by Blue Cross in the 1930s. Under experience rating, insurers avoid high-risk individuals and groups and increase premiums based upon illnesses experienced by enrollees. Experience rating weakens the ability of health insurance to share risk across a large risk pool of healthy and sick individuals.

Favorable risk selection: This is the process by which insurers screen potential enrollees according to health status, avoiding higher-risk sick individuals and groups in favor of healthier enrollees requiring less costly care—the opposite of adverse selection.

Federal poverty level (FPL): Annual income levels updated annually by the federal government defining poverty levels based on size of household. These are the guidelines for FFY 2015:

Family Size	100%	133%	200%
1	$11,670	$15,521	$23,340
2	$15,730	$20,920	$31,460
3	$19,790	$26,320	$39,580
4	$23,850	$31,720	$47,700

Fee-for-service (FFS): A common method of reimbursement for health services provided, such as by visit procedure, laboratory test or imaging study. Fees are often based on a fixed fee schedule or on more complex relative value scales. See also Resource-Based Relative Value Scale.

Fiscal Intermediary: Private insurers that have contracted with Medicare since the mid-1960s to administer hospitalization insurance under Part A of Medicare. Blue Cross has held most of these contracts over the years. In this capacity, insurers are empowered to make coverage and reimbursement decisions and to provide related administrative services

Formulary: Lists of drugs updated at regular intervals which can be prescribed by physicians for enrollees in specific health plans. Formulary development is a contentious area, with the pharmaceutical industry arguing for wider coverage lists while health plans strive to balance cost, efficacy, and safety issues against patients' access to medically necessary medications.

Gross domestic product (GDP): An economic indicator that measures the total output of everything produced by all the people and companies in a given country from year to year.

Guaranteed issue: This is typically opposed by the private health insurance industry because of the likelihood of adverse selection. The Affordable Care Act gives consumers new protections by banning insurers from denial of coverage because of pre-existing conditions.

Global budgets: These are annual negotiated budgets under single-payer national health insurance that will cover all costs of a hospital or other health care facility on an annual global basis.

Health exchanges: These were established under the ACA, for participating states or the federal government to provide a marketplace where consumers can shop for health plans that meet their pocket book and needs.

Health maintenance organization (HMO): HMOs are organizations that provide a broad range of services, coordinated by primary care physicians on a prepaid basis for enrollees. The earliest HMOs were established in the 1940s and 1950s, such as Kaiser Permanente and Group Health Cooperative of Puget Sound. They are integrated systems where physicians are salaried and work only with that HMO. Later years have seen the emergence of mostly for-profit HMOs that are looser structures contracting with physicians in independent practices who agree to provide managed care on a capitation basis for a panel of patients.

Health savings account (HSA): These were authorized under the Medicare Prescription Drug, Improvement, and Modernization Act of 2003 (MMA) as part of an effort to contain health care costs by shifting more financial responsibility to consumers for their health care choices and decisions. Employer and employee contributions to an HSA are tax-free when accompanied by high-deductible insurance policies. While providing new investment opportunities for healthy individuals, HSAs provide little financial protection against the costs of serious illness.

High-deductible health insurance plans (HDHI): There has been a growing trend in recent years for insurers and employers to offer HDHI plans with high cost-sharing requirements and annual deductibles as high as $10,000. These policies are typically associated with health savings accounts and provide little coverage or security for people experiencing significant medical expenses.

High-risk pool: With the goal to help people who have been denied coverage in the individual market, high-risk pools have been established by many states with federal and state funding as a means of pooling risk with others facing the same problem. The Affordable Care Act provides additional support for these high-risk pools, but their experience has been mostly disappointing because of the costs involved.

Individual market: The individual market is much smaller than that of employer-sponsored insurance. Many people with significant health issues find it difficult to gain affordable coverage in the individual market. The Affordable Care Act helps to a certain degree, especially by eliminating insurers' denial of coverage because of pre-existing conditions and providing subsidies for eligible enrollees, but coverage remains unaffordable for some.

Limited benefit plan: These are policies being marketed by private insurers to employers and healthier people with restricted benefits and annual caps as low as $1,000 to $2,500.

Managed care: Although this term has often become ambiguous and unclear in common usage, it expresses a relatively new relationship between purchasers, insurers, and providers of care. To a variable extent, organizations that pay for patient care have also taken on the role of making decisions about patient care management. In practice, however, "managed care" is often more managed reimbursement than care, with the possibility of perverse financial incentives to skimp on necessary services. There are three basic types of managed care organizations—preferred provider organizations (PPOs), group and staff model HMOs, and independent practice associations (IPA) HMOs.

Medicaid: This is a federal-state health insurance program, enacted in 1965, that covers low-income people who meet variable and changing state eligibility requirements. Most elderly, disabled, and blind individuals who receive assistance through the federal Supplemental Security Income (SSI) program are covered under Medicaid, which is also the main payer of nursing home costs. Current budget deficits in federal and state budgets threaten this vital safety net program, which provides last-resort coverage for about one in six Americans, including one-fifth of all children in the U.S.

Medicaid coverage gap: This refers to the approximately five million people who would have qualified for expanded Medicaid under the ACA but who live in states that opted out of Medicaid expansion. They are lower-income, uninsured adults with incomes above Medicaid eligibility levels but below the federal poverty level, so that they cannot qualify for either Medicaid or subsidies through the health exchanges.

Medical loss ratio (MLR): The medical loss ratio is that part of the premium dollar spent by insurers on direct medical care. Private insurers typically try to keep their MLR below the 80 or 85 percent level required by the Affordable Care Act, but have found ways to game that requirement by including other non-patient care expenses under "direct medical care."

Medical necessity: An elusive but important term which is applied to treatments and health care services that can be judged on the basis of clinical evidence to be effective and indicated as essential medical care.

It is an ongoing challenge for health professionals, insurers, payers and policymakers to define medical necessity as part of coverage policy, made more difficult as costs are considered and as new treatments are brought into use.

Medical underwriting: This is the process used by health insurers to calculate higher premiums to be charged to individual or group applicants at higher risk of illness. Medical underwriting was considered unethical in the early years of private health insurance in this country, but became the industry norm after the 1960s and is typically based on annual review of claims experience. Although the ACA prohibits insurers from denying coverage based on pre-existing conditions, private insurers still have other ways to avoid higher-risk enrollees, such as by selective marketing and tiering of benefits.

Medicare: A federal health insurance program for the elderly and disabled enacted in 1965 that now covers about 54 million Americans age 65 and older as well as younger adults with permanent disabilities, including those with chronic kidney failure. Traditional (Original) Medicare covers about one-half of beneficiaries' health care expenses, and accounts for about one-fifth of personal national health expenditures. There are four components of Medicare today:

> Part A: Hospitalization insurance
> Part B: Supplementary medical insurance
> Part C: Private Medicare plans, now Medicare Advantage
> Part D: Prescription drug coverage, starting in 2006.

Medicare Advantage: Private health plans authorized by Medicare legislation in 2003 as the sequel to Medicare + Choice programs. Most are HMOs, though many are preferred provider organizations (PPOs).

Medigap: These are private supplemental plans, available to people that already have Medicare Parts A and B, that help to cover some costs that Medicare does not cover, such as co-payments, coinsurance and deductibles. Medigap policies generally do not cover vision or dental care, hearing aids, eyeglasses or private duty nursing.

Monopsony purchasing: Purchasing of goods and services by a single buyer, such as bulk purchasing of prescription drugs by the Veterans Administration using the leverage of its population to obtain discounted prices from drug manufacturers.

National health insurance (NHI): A national health insurance program that would provide universal coverage to the entire U.S. population for necessary health care. It would be a single-payer system, government-financed with a private delivery system. Through simplified administration, it would provide more efficiency and cost containment than the current multi-payer market-based system while offering new opportunities to improve accountability and quality assurance within the system.

Network providers and hospitals: This designation is used by ACOs, HMOs and PPOs to indicate providers within networks of providers and hospitals. Networks today are typically set up by insurers and ACOs as ways to reduce their costs, not to improve continuity or quality of patient care. Patients are often penalized by having to pay more outside of these networks in order to receive care by their physicians and hospitals of choice.

Overpayments: These are administratively set payments to Medicare Advantage plans in excess of fee-for-service payments under traditional Medicare. Since the early years of private Medicare plans, insurers have successfully entrenched the concept that they should be paid more by the federal government than traditional Medicare, leading more to their increased profits than service to patients.

Pay for performance (P4P): An umbrella term referring to various approaches intended to improve the quality, efficiency and value of health care. A number of Medicare demonstration projects have been carried out over the last ten years to test this concept, which has been incorporated into the ACA. So far, P4P initiatives have not been found to contain costs or improve the quality of care.

Pre-existing condition: In the process of medical underwriting as insurers evaluate applicants for coverage, medical conditions which pre-date the application are scrutinized as they relate to future health risks. In the past, they have been used by insurers to deny coverage or raise initial premiums if coverage is offered. This practice has been eliminated by the ACA.

Preferred provider organization (PPO): A kind of health plan wherein providers agree to accept set discounted fees in exchange for the practice-building opportunity of being listed as a "preferred provider." Many patients favor a PPO that includes their physicians to an arbitrary network that excludes their chosen providers.

Premium support: This is a strategy promoted by its supporters intended to limit the government's financial responsibility to Medicare beneficiaries by shifting from a defined benefit program to a defined contribution approach. Under premium support, the government would pay a set amount toward the cost of a plan, whether FFS. HMO, or PPO, with enrollees responsible for any price differences. See also voucher.

Resource-based relative value scale (RBRVS): This is a system by which fees for physicians are set for each service by estimating such factors as time, mental effort and judgment, and technical skill involved in each service. RBRVS was adopted by Medicare in the early 1990s with the hope to reduce the wide disparities in reimbursement of procedure-oriented specialist and primary care physicians, but has not succeeded in this effort.

Risk adjustment: A complex technical process intended to estimate the difference in health status and risk in populations enrolled in Medicare private plans compared to FFS Medicare. It is well documented that private plans attract healthier patients requiring less costly care than traditional Medicare through favorable risk selection. Risk adjustment techniques so far have been too crude to deal with this problem.

Risk pool: A group of people considered together in order to price their insurance coverage. The larger and more diverse the group in terms of health status, the more effective insurance can be in having healthier individuals share the higher costs of care of sicker individuals while assuring the most affordable insurance premiums for the entire group.

Quality assurance: A broad field that has developed over the years with the goal to improve the quality of clinical practice, reduce the rate of medical errors, and improve patient care outcomes. This is an ongoing and difficult challenge, with evidence-based clinical practice guidelines an integral part of the process.

Single-payer: A single national financing system that covers an entire population. Traditional Medicare in the U.S. is one example, as is the Veterans Administration for veterans' health care. The U.S. has had legislation put forward in Congress on a number of occasions, such as H.R. 676 today, that would enact such a system of universal health insurance for all Americans. But so far there has not been the political will to overcome the resistance of private corporate stakeholders in our current market-based system. See also NHI.

Socialized medicine: Socialized medicine refers to a publicly-financed government owned and operated health care delivery system. The National Health Service in England is one such example, with government ownership of hospitals and physicians as salaried employees. The V.A. in this country is another example. National health insurance, as an expanded and improved Medicare for All program coupled with a private delivery system, would in no way be socialized medicine.

Social insurance: Social insurance is compulsory, usually provided by a public agency, and spreads the financial risk of illness across an entire population, making its costs affordable to a large population. This in marked contrast to private insurance, which is voluntary, provided by private insurers (usually for-profit) which selectively enroll better risks, thereby making coverage unaffordable or otherwise unavailable to higher-risk individuals. Traditional Medicare has been a social insurance program over the last 50 years, but is threatened by further privatization.

Underinsurance: As the costs of health care continue to rise at rates several times the cost-of-living and median family incomes, fewer people can afford insurance with comprehensive benefits. It they can afford coverage at all, they find themselves challenged by high levels of cost-sharing. The Commonwealth Fund has defined underinsurance on the basis of the proportion of total family income spent on health care (i.e. more than 10 percent of income, more that 5 percent of income if below 200 percent of federal poverty level, or deductibles equal to or exceeding 5 percent of income).

Uninsurance: This term refers to the many millions of Americans who, despite some relief from the ACA, remain without any health insurance. This is a large and heterogeneous group, still about one in five of our population. A majority of the uninsured are employed but without affordable coverage or in part-time work without benefits. Many uninsured lose coverage with a recent job change, divorce, or death of a previously insured spouse, while others do not qualify for such public safety net programs as Medicaid.

Universal coverage: This term describes countries that provide health insurance to all citizens regardless of age, income, or health status. The U.S. is an outlier among advanced countries around the world in not having universal coverage while spending far more than any other country for health care.

Utilization management (UM): A cost containment strategy used by Medicare, Medicaid, and many private plans that monitors the clinical activities of physicians. Payments for some services are denied if considered by the payer to be unnecessary. Critics of this approach contend that UM is an unwarranted intrusion into the physician-patient relationship, involves a burdensome administrative hassle for caregivers, and doesn't save much money anyway.

Voucher: A grant of money for a specific purpose, such as for meals or transportation. Conservatives have promoted the idea of vouchers for years as a way to reduce the government's responsibility for Medicare costs. Vouchers would shift Medicare from a program with defined benefits to one of defined contributions by the government to Medicare beneficiaries. Critics see this approach as a threat to the integrity and viability of the Medicare program, by also opening the door to stepwise further reductions in the level of government funding.

Index

Affordable Care Act scorecard
  delays and retreats, 119–120
  dysfunctional state exchanges, 112–113
  health exchange delays and shortfalls,
    110–112
  insurer inadequate accountability, 116–
    117 (Figure 7.1)–119
  Medicaid inadequate access and
    coverage, 114–116
  narrowed networks and barriers, 106–109
  newly insured through exchanges,
    113–114
  primary care shortage, 109–110
  states opting out of Medicaid expansion,
    103
AFL opposition to compulsory health
  insurance, 8
aging population, chronic diseases in, 233
AHIP. See America's Health Insurance Plans
Allison, Bill, 75 (quote)
Alterman, Eric, description of Fox News, 80
ambulatory surgery centers (ASCs),
  55–56
American Academy of Cosmetic Surgery, 70
American Board of Internal Medicine
Foundation, 58
American College of Physicians, 58, 273
American Enterprise Institute, 276
American Health Security Act, 14, 279
American Hospital Association
  Medicare support, 69
  not-for-profit plans, 10–11
  as stakeholder, 12
American Legislative Exchange Council
  (ALEC), 276–277
American Medical Association (AMA)
  Council on Medical Education, 23
  membership, percent of physicians, 58
  opposition to universal health care since
    1917, 69
  position on ACA, 7
  reimbursement methods, 195
  Relative Value Scale Update Committee
    (RUC), 127–128
  social insurance committee statement in
    1917, 7
  as stakeholder, 12
  UCR reimbursement system, 38
American Medical Students Association
(AMSA), 58
American Psychiatric Association, 273
American Public Health Association (APHA),
  58, 273
Americans for Prosperity, 277
Americans for Stable Quality Care, 68

American Society for Bioethics and
Humanities, 58
American Society of Clinical Oncology
  (ASCO), 273
American Women's Medical Association
  (AWMA), 58
America's Health Insurance Plans (AHIP),
  67, 88, 178, 189
Andrews, Charles (Profit Fever), 14
Angell, Marcia, social medicine lecturer/
  author, 198, 225, 234
Anthem Blue Cross, insurer, 91, 130, 171
Anthem/Wellpoint, 172, 176
ARA Living Centers, 35
Arrow, Kenneth, 224
Avalere Health insurance company, 132,
  137, 192

B

Bain Capital, 49
Bankrate Health Insurance Pulse survey and
  study, 111, 175
Barsky, Arthur, observations on changing
  medical practice, 25
Baucus, Senator Max, "Baucus Bill," and
  conflicts of interest, 68, 72, 77–78,
  167
Baucus Eight incident, 77–78
Baylor University Hospital prepaid group
  hospital plan, 9
Bertolini, Mark, Aetna CEO, 131
Berwick, Don, P4P quote, 152
Beverly Enterprises, 35
Big Four corporate alliance, 66–67, 70, 71
  (Table 5.1), 73, 80
  challenges to health care reform, 87
  drug industry (PhRMA), 68, 71,
    73
  hospital industry, 68–69, 71
  insurance industry, 67–68, 71, 73
  with media, talk shows, writers, editors,
book publishers, 79, 80
  organized medicine, 69–70, 71
Blue Cross
  lawsuit by Consumer Watchdog, 107
  prototype and not-for-profit plans, 10–11,
    13, 23
  support for Medicare, 69
Blue Cross Blue Shield letter from president
Bernard Tresnowski, 291
Blue Shield of California, 172
brachytherapy, radiation therapy, 157
Brill, Steven, testimony before Senate
  Finance Committee, 129
Brown, Lawrence D., comment on privatized

About the Author

John Geyman, M.D. is professor emeritus of family medicine at the University of Washington School of Medicine in Seattle, where he served as Chairman of the Department of Family Medicine from 1976 to 1990. As a family physician with over 25 years in academic medicine, he has also practiced in rural communities for 13 years. He was the founding editor of *The Journal of Family Practice* (1973 to 1990) and the editor of *The Journal of the American Board of Family Practice* from 1990 to 2003. His most recent books are *Health Care in America: Can Our Ailing System Be Healed?* (Butterworth-Heinemann, 2002), *The Corporate Transformation of Health Care: Can the Public Interest Still Be Served?* (Springer Publishing Company, 2004), *Falling Through the Safety Net: Americans Without Health Insurance* (2005), *Shredding the Social Contract: The Privatization of Medicare* (2006),

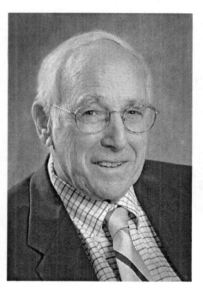

The Corrosion of Medicine: Can the Profession Reclaim its Moral Legacy? (2008), *Do Not Resuscitate: Why the Health Insurance Industry is Dying, and How We Must Replace It* (2008), *Hijacked: The Road to Single-payer in the Aftermath of Stolen Health Care Reform* (2010), *Breaking Point: How the Primary Care Crisis Endangers the Lives of Americans* (2011), *The Cancer Generation: Baby Boomers Facing a Perfect Storm*-Second Edition (2012), and *Health Care Wars: How Market Ideology and Corporate Power are Killing Americans* (2012), and *Souls on a Walk: An Enduring Love Story Unbroken by Alzheimer's* (2013).

Dr. Geyman served as president of Physicians for a National Health Program from 2005 to 2007 and is a member of the Institute of Medicine.